THE BODYBUILDING COOKBOOK
COLLECTION

CONTAINS OVER 200 DELICIOUS RECIPES TO BUILD MUSCLE, BURN FAT AND SAVE TIME

JASON FARLEY

Copyright

Legal Disclaimer

The information in the book is for educational purposes only. It is not medical advice and is not intended to replace the advice or attention of health-care professionals. Consult your physician before beginning or making any changes in your diet or exercise program. Specific medical advice should be obtained from a licensed health-care practitioner. Jason Farley and his associates will not assume any liability, nor be held responsible for any injury, illness or personal loss due to the utilization of any information contained herein.

CONTENTS

SECTION I:
THE BODYBUILDING COOKBOOK

SECTION II:
THE BODYBUILDING PALEO COOKBOOK

SECTION III:
THE VEGETARIAN BODYBUILDING COOKBOOK

SECTION IV
HOMEMADE PROTEIN SHAKES

SECTION V
DESSERTS

WELCOME

.

First off, I'd like to thank you for purchasing my book - The Bodybuilding Cookbook Collection. Within the following pages lies your complete nutritional toolkit for creating tasty muscle building meals that can be used to build muscle and burn fat!

Eating the right kind of foods is vital for anyone who wants to build muscle or get lean but it doesn't mean it has to be boring. So many athletes subject themselves to dull, bland meals, which becomes tedious, dull and repetitive over time. I created this book to teach you that it doesn't have to be that way. In this cookbook, you will find over 200 delicious, mouth-watering ways to build muscle and burn fat using all of my most loved recipes from my books – The Bodybuilding Cookbook, The Bodybuilding Paleo Cookbook and The Vegetarian Bodybuilding Cookbook.

Every recipe is easy to follow and easy to prepare. Each recipe also includes the exact amount of calories and the amount of protein, carbohydrates and fats you will get from each serving. The more higher calorie meals will be better suited to someone looking to build muscle and the lower calorie meals will be better suited to someone looking to burn fat. You won't need much equipment to make these recipes, at most a blender and a few pots and pans.

Without further ado, grab your apron and let's get cooking!

Enjoy your meals,

Jason Farley

MUSCLE IS WON OR LOST IN THE KITCHEN

Many experts feel that your nutritional habits make for up to 80% of the way your body looks. Every drip of sweat and effort you exude in the gym is wasted if your nutrition is not on point. If you want to build a substantial amount of muscle and strength or lose fat then you must fuel your body accordingly.

EATING FOR MUSCLE

To build muscle, you need to take in an excess of calories with the right nutrients to grow. If you don't eat enough, your body won't be able to fully repair the damage you cause by lifting weights, triggering you to plateau or even worse, lose muscle. However don't make the mistake most gym rats make by eating everything in sight, from pizzas to pop-tarts, as this is extremely unhealthy in the long-term. As you'll see from the upcoming recipes, eating the right foods doesn't have to be boring, bland or time–consuming.

EATING TO SHRED

To lose fat, you need to take in fewer calories than you expend. Again if you don't take in the right nutrients and foods, you will lose muscle. Losing fat generally requires you to be more precise which leads to many adopting the "Chicken, Rice and Broccoli diet," which is incredible boring, bland and usually leads to many people failing.

I created these recipes to escape the tedious, boring diets that many gym-goers subject themselves too and finally make dieting enjoyable.

THE FUNDAMENTAL PILLARS OF A MUSCLE BUILDING / FAT BURNING DIET

Before you ask, you won't need to be a qualified nutritionist to create your perfect diet. You just need to understand a few simple things:.

1. What Protein, Carbohydrates and Fats are and what they're used for.
2. How much to get of each and what foods to get them from.
3. How many calories you need to achieve your goals (Build Muscle or Burn Fat.)

WHAT IS PROTEIN?

Protein is used by your body for a number of processes from enzyme and hormone production to ensuring your immune system is working optimally. The reason why protein is so important in a muscle building diet is because protein is absolutely critical for muscle growth and repair. Working out and 'tearing down muscle' increases your body's demand for protein. As you build more and more muscle, the more protein your body will require to repair, grow and maintain that muscle. If you don't supply your body with enough protein, it will take it from your muscles causing muscle breakdown. Making sure you get enough protein is therefore of upmost importance in planning your diet.

WHAT ARE CARBOHYDRATES?

Carbohydrates get converted into glucose and then are used by your body for energy. There are two types of carbohydrates - simple and complex. Simple carbohydrates are foods like fruit, white rice and sugar. Complex carbohydrates are foods like sweet potatoes, brown rice and vegetables. Complex carbohydrates tend to be thought of as the better of the two. The difference between these types of carbohydrates is how long it takes the body to convert them into glucose. Simple carbohydrates are converted by your body quickly making them great for a fast source of energy however there is usually a fast decline after. It takes your body a lot longer to convert complex carbohydrates into glucose making them a much more sustaining source of energy. The reason so many people are afraid of carbohydrates is because whatever your body doesn't use gets moved into your fat stores. Carbohydrates however are not the enemy and are vital for your success.

WHAT ARE FATS?

Fats are vital for many of your bodily functions. They are needed for the production of many hormones in your body and they also help keep your brain and nervous system running optimally. They are also the most calorically dense out of the three macronutrients – every gram of fat contains 9 calories!
There are four types of fat: Monounsaturated, Polyunsaturated, Saturated and Trans-fatty acids. The only one you need to avoid is Trans-Fatty acids. These are fats that have been modified in a lab to ensure a longer shelf life. The body does not know what to do with them and therefore they can get into your cells and cause damage. They're most commonly found in packaged meals and used in many fried foods.

How much do you need of each? Well that depends on your goals!

TO BUILD MUSCLE, A GOOD PLACE TO START FROM IS:

Protein = 1.5 grams per pound of bodyweight Carbohydrates = 2 grams per pound of bodyweight
Fats = 0.5 grams per pound of bodyweight

> You want to be gaining about 0.5 – 1 pound a week. Any more than that and you will be gaining too much fat. If you find you aren't gaining weight, increase your calories by around 100-200 kcals each week until you reach the sweet spot. Alternatively if you're gaining too much, then you want to reduce your calories by around 100 – 200 each week.

TO MAINTAIN MUSCLE, A GOOD PLACE TO START FROM IS:

Protein= 1 gram per pound of bodyweight, Carbohydrates = 1 gram per pound of bodyweight
Fats = 0.5 grams per pound of bodyweight

TO LOSE WEIGHT, A GOOD PLACE TO START FROM IS:

Protein = 2 grams per pound of bodyweight, Carbohydrates = 0.5 grams per pound of bodyweight
Fats = 1 gram per pound of bodyweight

> You want to be losing about 1 – 2 pound a week. Any more than that and you risk losing that hard earned muscle. If you find you aren't losing weight, decrease your calories by around 100-200 kcals each week until you reach the sweet spot. Alternatively if you're losing too much, then you want to increase your calories by around 100 – 200 each week.

THE TOP COMMANDMENTS OF GOOD NUTRITION

What you put into your body will either make or break the results you get in the gym. These are rules you must live by if you want to be successful in your muscle building and fat loss pursuits.

1. HAVE PROTEIN WITH EVERY MEAL

Protein is vital to your success if building or maintaining muscle mass is your goal. Aim to have a least 1 source of quality protein with every meal. At a minimum, you must aim for at least 1 pound of protein per pound of bodyweight.

2. THERE MUST BE GREEN ON THE PLATE

Vegetables contain so many essential nutrients that you simply can't get anywhere else. Aim to have at least 1 serving of vegetables with every meal.

3. FAT IS NOT EVIL

Lets get one thing straight; fat will not make you fat. If you want to build muscle and burn fat, it's vital that you get enough. As we've established, healthy fats are needed for the production of many hormones in your body including testosterone. The only fats you need to avoid are trans fats.

4. DON'T RELY ON SUPPLEMENTS, EAT (REAL) FOOD

Supplements are meant to supplement your diet not make up the bulk of it. Aim to have at least 70% of your diet come from "real" food.

5. STICK TO SLOW DIGESTING CARBS MOST OF THE TIME (EXCEPT AROUND YOUR WORKOUTS)

Slow digesting carbohydrates ensure a steady supply of energy and have less of an impact on your blood sugar levels. Regular consumption of fast digesting carbs has been linked to an increased risk of diabetes, heart disease and obesity. However after training, you want to replace your depleted glycogen stores quickly as this can prevent your body becoming catabolic and keep you in a "muscle building" state. This is why you would want to consume a fast digesting carbohydrate after your workout.

6. DRINK WATER AND LOTS OF IT

It is absolutely essential to drink enough water. When you don't get enough, performance can be severely affected. Therefore try to get in about 3 – 4 litres of pure, clean water per day.

BREAKFAST

It's the most important meal of the day. Your parents told you. Your teachers told you. And now you know it. How can you expect not to have a total burn out, or beat your PB, or even have the energy to get your ass off the sofa if you haven't fuelled the machine? You can't. So use these quick, easy and tasty recipes to get you going. And no, it's not all raw eggs…

MASS BUILDING
SWEET POTATO PANCAKES

Start your day with this quick and easy, delicious protein packed pancake recipe. It contains all the right ingredients to keep you going and more than enough protein for your muscles to feast on!

CALORIES PER SERVING: 451

PROTEIN: 38G

CARBS: 74G

FAT: 9G

SERVES 1

1 medium sized sweet potato

1 egg

4 egg whites

100g of fat-free Greek yogurt

40g of oats

1 tsp cinnamon

1 tsp vanilla extract

Handful of diced strawberries

Handful of blueberries

1 tsp of honey

HOW TO MAKE:

Rinse sweet potato under cold water for a couple of seconds and then pierce it with a fork several times and place it in the microwave until soft (about 8 minutes).

After let it cool down before removing all skin with a knife.

Put the oats into a blender and blend until they are a fine powder, then place into a bowl.

Place the sweet potato in the blender and blend until smooth, and then mix with the powdered oats.

Add the egg, egg whites, vanilla, cinnamon, honey and yogurt and stir well. This is now your pancake batter.

Spray a pan with cooking spray and place over medium heat. Pour roughly a quarter of the batter into the pan and cook for 1-2 minutes.

Flip the pancake and cook for another 30 seconds. Once done, remove your tasty pancake and top with the berries. Use the same method for the rest of your batter.

BRAWNY BREAKFAST BURRITO

Add a bit spice to your life with this Mexican inspired burrito. Contains great sources of protein, healthy fats and fibre to ensure you're building muscle the lean way.

CALORIES PER SERVING: 302

PROTEIN: 25G

CARBS: 19G

FAT: 16G

SERVES 1

2 eggs

50ml of low fat milk

25g of black beans

50g of low fat cheese

Handful of chopped red peppers

1tsp of chopped coriander

1tbsp of salsa

½ a tsp of cumin

HOW TO MAKE:

Add the milk, eggs and cumin to a bowl and whisk together.

Spray pan with cooking spray and place over medium heat. Add the mixture to the pan.

After roughly 2 – 3 minutes, add the low fat cheese, chopped red peppers and black beans to the omelette.

Once added fold the omelette in half and let it cook through (1-2 minutes).

Remove from pan and serve with the salsa and coriander.

SUPER SCRAMBLED
TURKEY BACON EGGS ON TOAST

Mix up your boring egg based breakfasts with this delicious recipe. Eggs are a great source of complete protein as they contain all eight amino acids.

CALORIES PER SERVING: 299

PROTEIN: 22G

CARBS: 35G

FAT: 8G

SERVES 2

6 egg whites

3 slices of turkey bacon

2 slices of Ezekiel bread

Handful of chopped onion

Handful of chopped peppers

Handful of chopped white mushrooms

1tsp of garlic powder

1tsp of dried parsley

1tsp of olive oil

HOW TO MAKE:

Spray pan with cooking spray and place over medium/high heat. Add the chopped onions, chopped yellow peppers and white mushrooms and cook until soft.

In a different pan, cook the turkey bacon.

Add the egg whites and garlic powder to the pan with the veggies and 1tsp of olive oil and scramble until the eggs become firm.

Toast the Ezekiel bread.

Break up the turkey bacon and add to the scrambled eggs

Plate up and serve scrambled eggs and turkey bacon on bread, sprinkled with the fresh parsley.

Add salt and pepper as required.

BANANA AND ALMOND MUSCLE OATMEAL

If you're in a hurry, this recipe is great. It takes around 5 minutes to make and still has the right macro-nutrients to make this a healthy and sustaining meal.

CALORIES PER SERVING: 523

PROTEIN: 32G

CARBS: 60G

FAT: 15G

HOW TO MAKE:

Throw the oats and low fat milk into a large bowl and place in the micro-wave for two minutes.

Add the diced banana, peanut butter, whey protein and chopped almonds to the oats and mix in.

SERVES 1

50 grams of rolled oats

200ml of low fat milk

1 scoop of whey protein (vanilla or chocolate)

Handful of chopped almonds

1tsp of organic peanut butter

1 diced banana

PROTEIN
POWERED PANCAKES

If you're not a fan of sweet potato, then these are a great alternative. Lots of protein and quick and easy to make.

CALORIES PER SERVING: 337

PROTEIN: 27G

CARBS: 33G

FAT: 9G

MAKES 5 PANCAKES

6 egg whites

40g of rolled oats

1 tsp flaxseed oil

1 tsp of cinnamon

1 tsp of stevia

HOW TO MAKE:

Put the oats and all the other ingredients into a blender and blend. This is now your pancake batter.

Spray pan with cooking spray and place over medium heat.

Pour roughly 1/5 of the pancake batter into the pan and cook for 1-2 minutes. Flip the pancake and cook for another 30 seconds.

Once done, remove your tasty pancake.

Use the same method for the rest of your batter.

TURKEY
MUSCLE OMELETTE

If you're looking for a protein packed, low carb meal for breakfast then this is it. Contains 26 grams of protein and only 5 grams of carbs.

CALORIES PER SERVING: 358

PROTEIN: 26G

CARBS: 5G

FAT: 21G

SERVES 2

150g of chopped or minced turkey

3 eggs

Handful of baby spinach

Handful of kale

1 tbsp of olive oil

25g of low fat cheese

HOW TO MAKE:

Crack the eggs into a bowl and whisk.

Grab a pan and heat half the oil on a medium heat, then add the turkey, kale and cheese and cook for 5-6 minutes.

In a different pan, heat the rest of the olive oil and then add the eggs and cook for around 4 minutes.

Add the turkey mix into the pan with the eggs and sprinkle some baby spinach on top, then fold the omelette in half.

Cook for another 2-3 minutes.

Plate up and serve.

AESTHETIC
ASPARAGUS FRITTATA

A high protein, low carb breakfast. Great for those looking to minimize their carb intake

CALORIES PER SERVING: 349

PROTEIN: 23G

CARBS: 8G

FAT: 25G

SERVES 3

300g of chopped asparagus

½ broccoli (florets only)

8 eggs

Handful of chopped parsley

1 tsp of chives

1 tbsp of olive oil

100ml of low fat milk

Salt and pepper

HOW TO MAKE:

Crack the eggs into a bowl, add the milk and some salt and pepper and whisk.

Get a covered skillet and steam the broccoli over a medium heat for 4-5 minutes. Set to one side.

Next, in the same skillet, heat the oil. Add the chopped asparagus, chopped parsley and chives into the skillet and cook for around 2-3 minutes on a medium heat.

Add the egg mixture, along with the broccoli into the skillet and cover the skillet evenly.

Cook for around 3-4 minutes or until the eggs are set right through

Take the skillet and place under the grill for around 2 minutes or until the top is golden (optional).

Plate up and serve.

POWER
PROTEIN WAFFLES

Who said waffles are unhealthy? My waffle recipes are packed full of protein and without the guilt on the side!

CALORIES PER SERVING: 314

PROTEIN: 37G

CARBS: 28G

FAT: 5G

HOW TO MAKE:

Add all the ingredients into a blender and blend.

Add the mixture to a waffle iron and bake.

SERVES 2

4 eggs whites

1 scoop of vanilla protein powder

40g of rolled oats

1 tsp of baking powder

½ tsp of stevia

SCRAMBLED EGGS WITH SPINACH

Tasty, quick and easy breakfast packed full of protein!

CALORIES PER SERVING: 282

PROTEIN: 23G

CARBS: 15G

FAT: 15G

SERVES 2

3 eggs

5 egg whites

1 cup of baby spinach

50g of grated low fat cheese

Handful of chopped onion

Handful of chopped red peppers

1 tsp of olive oil

HOW TO MAKE:

Spray pan with cooking spray and place over medium/high heat.

Add the chopped onions, chopped red peppers and cook until soft.

Add the egg and egg whites to the pan with the veggies with 1tsp of olive oil and scramble until the eggs become firm.

Sprinkle the baby spinach leaves and cheese over the eggs.

Plate up and serve scrambled eggs.

Add salt and pepper as required.

CHICKEN AND POULTRY

Chicken breast and eggs. The first things you might be mistaken to think you have to subject yourself to for breakfast, lunch and dinner for the rest of your muscle-building life. But there is so much more out there within the chicken and poultry meal options. We all know chicken is great – it's low in fat and high in protein and we all know it's tasty so read on and find out how chicken and other poultry members can be exciting and effective in your meal-plan diary.

QUICK AND EASY
GRILLED CHICKEN WRAPS

These are quick to prepare and full of protein to build muscle and burn fat. Ideal for lunchboxes!

CALORIES PER SERVING: 437

PROTEIN: 48G

CARBS: 39G

FAT: 10G

HOW TO MAKE:

Get 1 whole-wheat tortilla and spread the low-fat mayonnaise across the centre.

Add the grilled chicken, cucumber, spinach leaves and red pepper to the mayonnaise and roll the tortilla up.

Repeat the process with the last tortilla.

SERVES 1

2 whole-wheat tortilla wraps

150g of chopped grilled chicken

1tsp of low-fat mayonnaise

Handful of baby spinach leaves

1/2 a sliced cucumber

1/2 chopped red pepper

ANABOLIC
JERK CHICKEN AND BROWN RICE

Add a little spice to your life with this traditional Caribbean dish. Packed full of protein and slow releasing carbohydrates to keep to you growing.

CALORIES PER SERVING: 516

PROTEIN: 32G

CARBS: 76G

FAT: 33G

SERVES 1

100g of chicken thighs or breast	½ of dried thyme
½ tsp of ground allspice	1 chopped onion
½ tsp of black pepper	2 scotch bonnet chillies
½ tsp of nutmeg	1/2 chopped red pepper
½ tsp of cinnamon	60g of brown rice
½ tsp of sage	1 tsp of olive oil
½ tsp of dried thyme	
1 clove of garlic	

HOW TO MAKE:

To make the jerk paste, add the allspice, nutmeg, sage, cinnamon, dried thyme, garlic, red pepper, black pepper, onion, olive oil and scotch bonnet chillies to the blender and blend until it's a puree.

Rub the paste over the chicken breasts and leave them for at least one hour to marinade.

Add the chicken breasts to the grill and grill them for roughly 10-12 minutes per side or until they are cooked through. Put to one side once cooked.

Meanwhile add 300ml of cold water to a pot and heat until the water is boiling. Once boiling, add the rice and leave for 20 minutes.

Drain the rice and serve with the chicken.

LAZY CHICKEN
AND EGG STIR FRY

This meal is quick to prepare and contains two great protein sources to build muscle and burn fat.

CALORIES PER SERVING: 409

PROTEIN: 46G

CARBS: 89G

FAT: 20G

SERVES 1

100g of chopped chicken breast

2 eggs

100g of brown rice

2 tsp of chinese five spice

100g of Mixed frozen veg

HOW TO MAKE:

Add 300ml of cold water to a pot and heat until the water is boiling. Once boiling, add the rice and leave for 20 minutes. Drain the rice and place to one side.

Heat a pan on a medium heat and add the chopped chicken and spices.

Stir-fry for roughly 5 minutes.

While the chicken is cooking, boil or steam the frozen veg for 5 minutes until cooked and beat the eggs in a separate bowl.

Add the rice and beaten eggs to the pan with the chicken and stir until the eggs start to scramble 3-4 minutes.

Finally add the veg to the pan and stir for a further 2-3 minutes

Plate up and serve.

POWER
PESTO CHICKEN PASTA

Great protein packed pasta dish to mix things up!

CALORIES PER SERVING: 550

PROTEIN: 25G

CARBS: 30G

FAT: 19G

SERVES 2

200g of chopped grilled chicken breast

100g of whole-wheat pasta

1 tbsp of pesto

A pinch of black pepper

Handful of basil

Handful of spinach

Handful of rocket

Handful of pine nuts

Handful of diced tomatoes

2 tbsp of olive oil

HOW TO MAKE:

Heat a large pan of water on high until it boils.

Add the whole-wheat pasta and leave until the water returns to boiling point.

Reduce the heat until the water simmers. Leave the whole-wheat pasta to cook for around 10 minutes.

Get a bowl and add the pesto, olive oil and black pepper and mix together.

Add the chopped chicken breast, pine nuts, tomatoes and herbs to the mixture.

Drain the pasta and fold the mix into the pan until the pasta is covered.

MUSCLE
MOROCCAN CHICKEN CASSEROLE

This meal is quick to prepare and contains two great protein sources to build muscle and burn fat.

CALORIES PER SERVING: 409

PROTEIN: 46G

CARBS: 89G

FAT: 20G

SERVES 1

4 chicken breasts

1 tsp of ground cumin

1 tsp of paprika

1 tbsp of olive oil

1 chopped onion

350g of canned chopped tomatoes

2 tbsp harissa paste

1 tbsp honey

2 medium thickly sliced courgettes

400g of drained and rinsed chickpeas

A pinch of salt and pepper

HOW TO MAKE:

Sprinkle salt, pepper, paprika and the ground cumin over the chicken breasts.

Then grab a large pan and add the olive oil and heat on a medium heat.

Add the chicken and onions to the pan and cook the chicken for roughly four minutes per side.

Pour the chopped tomatoes into the pan along with 200ml of water and add the honey, harissa, courgettes and chickpeas and stir the ingredients together.

Bring the mix to a simmer and then leave to cook for around 15 minutes.

Plate up and serve.

BRAWNY CHICKEN & CHORIZO JAMBALAYA

A very tasty muscle-building recipe, inspired from Cajun cuisine. Contains a good helping of protein and slow releasing carbs to keep you burning fat and building muscle.

CALORIES PER SERVING: 286

PROTEIN: 30G

CARBS: 61G

FAT: 14G

SERVES 4

2 chopped chicken breasts

1 chopped onion

1 chopped red pepper

2 crushed garlic cloves

100g chorizo, sliced

1 tbsp Cajun seasoning

250g brown rice

1 tbsp olive oil

350g of tinned chopped tomatoes

350ml chicken stock

HOW TO MAKE:

Grab a large pan and add the olive oil and heat on a medium heat.

Add the chicken and brown for around 8 minutes. Place to one side.

Add the onion to the pan and fry until tender. Get the garlic, chorizo, Cajun seasoning and red pepper and add to the pan and cook for around 5 minutes.

Add the brown rice along with the chopped tomatoes, chicken and chicken stock to the pan. Cover the pan and let simmer for around 25 minutes or until the rice is soft.

SPICY
CHICKEN TRAY-BAKE

A very simple to make chicken recipe that tastes great and contains all the necessary muscle building nutrients.

CALORIES PER SERVING: 276

PROTEIN: 40G

CARBS: 14G

FAT: 7G

SERVES 4

4 skinless chicken breasts

3 tbsp harissa paste

250g of low-fat natural yogurt

1 small, chopped and peeled butter-nut squash

2 chopped red onions

1 tbsp olive oil

HOW TO MAKE:

Pre-heat oven (375°F/190 °C/Gas Mark 5).

Add 3 tbsp of yogurt and 2 tbsp of the harissa to a bowl and mix together. Coat the chicken breast with the mixture and leave to one side.

Add the onions, chopped butternut squash, 1 tbsp of harissa and 2 tbsp of olive oil to a tray and place in the oven and cook for around 10 minutes.

Take the tray out of the oven and add the chicken breast to the tray. Place back in the oven and cook for around 20 minutes until the chicken is cooked right through.

Plate up and serve with the leftover yogurt.

HEALTHY
TURKEY BURGERS

Get your burger fix with this healthy turkey alternative.

CALORIES PER SERVING: 362

PROTEIN: 38G

CARBS: 39G

FAT: 7G

SERVES 4

500g of mince turkey

1 onion, finely chopped

1 chopped romaine lettuce

4 wholemeal buns

2 diced tomatoes

1 crushed garlic clove

1 lemon

3 tbsp grated parmesan

Chopped parsley

3 tbsp low-fat Greek yogurt

HOW TO MAKE:

Pre-heat oven (375°F/190 °C/Gas Mark 5).

In a bowl, add the crushed garlic, 2 tbsp of parmesan and parsley.

Cut the lemon in half and squeeze the lemon juice over the ingredients.

Mix all the ingredients together.

Add the ingredients to the minced turkey along with the onion and mix them together.

Using your hands, mould the mince mixture into 4 burgers and place on a tray and then cook for around 20 minutes or until the burgers have cooked right through.

While the burgers are cooking, cut open the whole-wheat buns and mix the yogurt with the lettuce. Add the burgers to the buns along with the yogurt-lettuce mixture and tomatoes.

TURKEY MEATBALL FIESTA

Healthy turkey meatballs with added oats to keep you building muscle and burning fat.

CALORIES PER SERVING: 315

PROTEIN: 35G

CARBS: 23G

FAT: 10G

SERVES 4

500g of turkey mince	1 tsp olive oil	3 tsp chipotle chilli paste
50g porridge oats	1 chopped red onion	300ml chicken stock
2 chopped spring onions	2 chopped garlic cloves	400g of canned chopped tomatoes
1 tsp ground cumin	1 large chopped yellow pepper	400g of drained black beans
1 tsp coriander	1 tsp ground cumin	
Handful of chopped coriander		1 avocado, stoned, peeled and chopped

HOW TO MAKE:

Add the mince to a bowl with the oats, chopped spring onions, spices and coriander and mix together.

Mould the mince mixture into 12 small 'meatballs' using your hands.

Add some olive oil to the pan on a medium heat; add the meatballs and cook them until golden.

Take them from the pan and leave to one side.

Add the onion, chopped pepper and chopped garlic to the pan and cook until tender.

Add the chilli paste and ground cumin and chicken stock to the pan and stir well. Then add the meatballs back into the pan.

Cover and cook on a low/medium heat for around 10 minutes.

Add the tomatoes and black beans to the pan and cook uncovered for around 2-3 minutes.

Serve with the chopped avocado and coriander.

ANABOLIC
RATATOUILLE CHICKEN

A tasty low-carb chicken recipe to keep you building muscle and burning fat.

CALORIES PER SERVING: 324

PROTEIN: 38G

CARBS: 10G

FAT: 15G

SERVES 4

4 chicken breasts

1 chopped onion,

2 chopped red peppers

1 courgette, cut into chunks

1 small aubergine, cut into chunks

4 chopped tomatoes

4 tbsp of olive oil

A pinch of salt and pepper

HOW TO MAKE:

Pre-heat oven (375°F/190 °C/Gas Mark 5).

Add all the vegetables and the tomatoes to a tray and drizzle with 3 tbsp. olive oil.

Place the chicken breasts over the vegetables and season with the remaining tbsp of olive oil and some salt and pepper.

Place the tray in the oven and cook for around 30 minutes.

Plate up and serve

BRAWNY
CHICKEN CHASSEUR

A classic, tasty chicken dish that's packed with protein and low carbs.

CALORIES PER SERVING: 242

PROTEIN: 50G

CARBS: 5G

FAT: 3G

SERVES 4

8 chopped rashers of turkey bacon

4 chopped chicken breasts

200g of baby mushrooms

1 tbsp plain flour

400g of canned chopped tomatoes

1 beef stock cube

Worcestershire sauce

Handful of chopped parsley

Olive oil

HOW TO MAKE:

Heat the olive oil on a medium heat in a shallow saucepan and add the turkey bacon and cook for 4-5 minutes until it starts to brown.

Add the chopped chicken breasts and cook for around 5 minutes until golden. Increase the heat to high and add the baby mushrooms for 2 minutes. Add the flour and stir in until a paste starts to form.

Add the canned chopped tomatoes and beef stock cube to the saucepan and cook for around 10 minutes.

Then add the parsley and Worcestershire sauce to the pan, stir in and then serve.

AESTHETIC
TOMATO AND OLIVE PAN-FRIED CHICKEN

A tasty chicken dish that's sure to satisfy your hunger and nutritional needs.

CALORIES PER SERVING: 334

PROTEIN: 39G

CARBS: 8G

FAT: 19G

SERVES 2

2 Chicken breasts

1 chopped onion,

2 chopped garlic cloves

400g of canned chopped tomatoes

1 tbsp balsamic vinegar

6 chopped green olives

300ml chicken stock

2 tbsp olive oil

Handful of basil leaves

A pinch of salt and pepper

HOW TO MAKE:

Heat olive oil on a medium heat in a pan.

Sprinkle some salt and pepper over the chicken and then place the chicken in the pan and cook for roughly 10 minutes, or until the chicken has cooked right through..

Add the onion to the pan and turn the chicken over and cook for another 4 – 5 minutes. Remove the chicken from the pan and place to one side.

Add the garlic to the pan and continue to cook the onions until tender.

Add the chopped tomatoes, olives, chicken stock and balsamic vinegar to the pan with most of the basil leaves and turn down the heat, simmering for around 8 minutes.

Place the chicken back into the pan, cover and simmer for a further 5 minutes

Plate up and serve with the remaining basil as a garnish.

CHICKEN
BRAWN BURGER

Another great healthy burger alternative! Quick and easy to make if you're strapped for time. Contains a good helping of protein to keep you anabolic.

CALORIES PER SERVING: 458

PROTEIN: 50G

CARBS: 38G

FAT: 12G

SERVES 1

1 chicken breast

1 tbsp low fat mayonnaise

1 chopped red onion

1 chopped lettuce

1 slice of low-fat cheddar

1 whole wheat burger bun

1 tsp of chopped jalapeno

Olive oil

HOW TO MAKE:

Heat olive oil on a medium heat in a griddle pan.

Cover the chicken breast with some salt and pepper and add to the pan and cook for around 5 minutes. Turn it over and cook for a further 5 minutes.

Add the slice of cheddar to the top of the chicken. Cook chicken for another 8 minutes or until chicken is cooked right through.

Remove chicken from pan and place to one side.

Cut open the roll and add the chicken, onions, mayonnaise, lettuce and chopped jalapeno

.

TASTY
TURKEY BAGEL

Quick and easy great recipe, ideal for lunch or post-workout. Contains lots of protein to keep you growing.

CALORIES PER SERVING: 336

PROTEIN: 21G

CARBS: 64G

FAT: 1G

HOW TO MAKE:

Cut the whole-wheat bagel in half and then add each half to the toaster.

Add the turkey breast, chopped tomato, cucumber, spinach and rocket to the bagel.

Serve on the go or at home!

SERVES 1

2 thick deli turkey breast slices

1 whole-wheat bagel

Handful of baby spinach

Handful of rocket

1 chopped tomato

¼ sliced cucumber

DICED
CHICKEN WITH EGG NOODLES

Mix things up with this tasty recipe. Contains the right amount of protein, carbs and fats to meet your goals.

CALORIES PER SERVING: 322

PROTEIN: 30G

CARBS: 31G

FAT: 8G

SERVES 2

150g of chopped chicken breast

50g of egg noodles

1 grated carrot

2 tbsp of fresh orange juice

1 tsp of sesame seeds

3 tsp of soy sauce

1 tsp of rapeseed oil

1 chopped ginger

100g of sugar snap peas

HOW TO MAKE:

Heat 1 tsp rapeseed oil on a medium heat in pan.

Cook the chopped chicken breast for about 10-15 minutes or until cooked through.

While cooking the chicken, place the noodles in a pot of boiling water for about 5 minutes.

In a bowl, mix together the ginger, sesame seeds, soy sauce, 1 tsp rapeseed oil and orange juice.

Once chicken is cooked and noodles are cooked and drained, add the chicken, noodles, carrot and peas to the dressing and mix

HONEY
GLAZED GROWTH CHICKEN

Mix things up with this sweet and tempting chicken recipe

CALORIES PER SERVING: 195

PROTEIN: 37G

CARBS: 9G

FAT: 2G

SERVES 2

2 chicken breasts with skin

½ lemon

1 tbsp honey

1 tbsp dark soy sauce

A pinch of salt and pepper

HOW TO MAKE:

Pre-heat oven (375°F/190 °C/Gas Mark 5).

Place the chicken breast on a baking dish and add a sprinkle of salt and pepper.

Get a bowl and squeeze the lemon juice in and add the honey and soy sauce. Mix the ingredients together and cover the chicken breasts with it.

Place the squeezed lemon in between the chicken breasts and place the dish into the oven and cook for around 30 minutes on until fully cooked through.

MIGHTY
MEXICAN CHICKEN STEW

Spice things up with this classic Mexican chicken stew. Packed full of protein from the chicken as well as the quinoa!

CALORIES PER SERVING: 464

PROTEIN: 51G

CARBS: 53G

FAT: 4G

SERVES 4

4 skinless chicken breasts

140g quinoa

400g of drained pinto beans

1 tbsp olive oil

1 chopped onion

2 chopped red peppers

3 tbsp chipotle paste

800g of tinned chopped tomatoes

2 chicken stock cubes

Handful of chopped coriander

1 lime

HOW TO MAKE:

Heat olive oil on a medium heat in a deep pan and add the onion and peppers and cook for 2-3 minutes.

Then add the chipotle paste and the tinned chopped tomatoes.

Add the chicken breast and add just enough water to cover the chicken by 1cm and then bring down the heat to let the mixture simmer. Cook for around 20 minutes until the chicken is cooked right through.

Add boiling water to a separate saucepan along with stock cubes. Pour in the quinoa and heat for around 12 minutes.

Add the pinto beans and cook for a further 3 minutes. Drain the quinoa and add in the coriander and squeeze the lime juice in - mix and place to one side.

Serve the chicken with the quinoa and cover with the tomato sauce from the pan.

SPICY
CAJUN CHICKEN WITH GUACAMOLE

Tasty low fat, low carb chicken recipe. Contains a generous amount of protein to keep you building muscle and burning fat.

CALORIES PER SERVING: 190

PROTEIN: 34G

CARBS: 2G

FAT: 5G

SERVES 4

4 chicken breasts

1 tbsp paprika

1 tsp dried onion flakes

¼ tsp cayenne pepper

2 tsp dried thyme

Salt

Pepper

1 tbsp olive oil

200g of guacamole

HOW TO MAKE:

Get a bowl and add the cayenne pepper, dried thyme, paprika, salt, pepper and onion flakes and mix together.

Get the chicken and cut two deep scores on each breast. Rub the oil onto the chicken then cover the breasts with the spices.

Add the chicken to the grill and cook for around 8 minutes each side or until completely cooked through.

Serve chicken with the guacamole

MUSCLE
CHICKEN CACCIATORE

An Italian inspired, delicious, low fat, low carb chicken recipe. Contains a liberal amount of protein to keep you building muscle and burning fat.

CALORIES PER SERVING: 172

PROTEIN: 33G

CARBS: 6G

FAT: 2G

SERVES 4

4 chicken breasts

1 chopped onion

2 sliced garlic cloves

Salt

Pepper

1 tsp olive oil

400g of tinned chopped tomatoes

2 tbsp chopped rosemary leaves

Handful of basil leaves

HOW TO MAKE:

Pre-Heat oven (375°F/190 °C/Gas Mark 5).

Heat oil in a pan on a medium heat and add the onion and garlic and cook until soft.

Pour in the chopped tomatoes, rosemary, salt and pepper and cook for around 15 minutes until the mixture has become thicker.

Spread the mixture over the chicken; place the chicken on a tray and transfer to the oven. Leave in the oven for 20 minutes until the chicken is cooked right through. Sprinkle the basil over the chicken and serve

RED MEAT AND PORK

I've teamed pork with red meat because it has every bit as much macho power! Pork doesn't have to be dry and fatty it can be delicious with the recipes to follow. Red meat speaks for itself in the muscle building world – a slab of steak comes to anybody's mind when they are trying to get big! Hopefully from the next section I can provide you with alternative dishes to fill you up with iron, protein and much more!

BRAWNY
BEEF SANDWICHES

It's a hell of a lot cheaper to make your own sandwiches and a lot healthier than the shop-bought ones too. This brawny sandwich provides plenty of protein to keep you anabolic.

CALORIES PER SERVING: 545

PROTEIN: 43G

CARBS: 64G

FAT: 10G

HOW TO MAKE:

Get 2 slices of bread.

Add 2 slices of deli beef, 1 tsp of mustard, ½ a sliced cucumber, spinach and a pinch of black pepper to the slice and make a sandwich.

Repeat the process with the rest of the ingredients.

Simple.

SERVES 1

4 slices of deli beef

4 slices of whole-wheat bread

2 tsp of mustard

Handful of baby spinach leaves

1/2 a sliced cucumber

A pinch of black pepper

ANABOLIC PORK SOUP

This soup is quick to prepare and full of protein to build muscle and burn fat.

CALORIES PER SERVING: 297

PROTEIN: 21G

CARBS: 13G

FAT: 17G

SERVES 4

400g diced pork steaks

600ml chicken stock

1 tbsp soy sauce

2 tsp Chinese five-spice powder

25 ginger finely chopped

200g pack of baby spinach

1 tsp of chopped red chilli,

200g of rice noodles

Handful of chopped spring onions

HOW TO MAKE:

Get a large saucepan and add all the ingredients except for the spring onions and noodles. Cover the pan and bring to a simmer on a medium heat.

Without letting the ingredients boil, leave to cook for around 8-10 minutes.

While cooking the pork, place the rice noodles in a pot of boiling water for about 5 minutes and then drain.

Drain and place the noodles in a bowl and add the pork and greens over the noodles. Sprinkle the spring onions over the dish and serve.

POWER
PORK FRUIT TRAY

This dish is absolutely delicious and one of my favourite pork recipes. Contains a good helping of protein and is low on carbs for those of you who are shredding!

CALORIES PER SERVING: 335

PROTEIN: 42G

CARBS: 12G

FAT: 14G

SERVES 4

4 pork steaks

1 tbsp olive oil

2 diced red onions

2 chopped large pears

Small handful of rosemary

50g diced blue cheese

1 diced couchette

Handful of pine nuts

HOW TO MAKE:

Get a large pan and heat the olive oil on a medium heat.

Add the courgette, red onions, chopped pears, salt and pepper.

Fry for around 6 minutes until the veg starts to caramelise.

Pre-heat the Grill.

Get a cooking tray and transfer the ingredients along with the rosemary sprigs to the tray. Sprinkle some salt and pepper over the pork steaks and place them in the tray.

Place the tray in the oven and grill for around 10-15 minutes or until cooked right through, turning the pork steaks half way through. Add the cheese and pine nuts and let the cheese melt for a further 4-5 minutes.

Plate up and serve.

MUSCLE BUILDING
STEAK & SWEET POTATO FRIES

A great, healthy alternative to regular steak and chips. Contains a good helping of protein and slow releasing carbs.

CALORIES PER SERVING: 418

PROTEIN: 29G

CARBS: 39G

FAT: 15G

SERVES 4

100g of sirloin steak

200g of sweet potatoes cut into chips

1 tbsp olive oil

1 chopped red onion

1 bag of pre-washed salad

1 tbsp of balsamic vinegar

A pinch of black pepper

HOW TO MAKE:

Pre-Heat oven (375°F/190 °C/Gas Mark 5).

Get a baking tray, spread the chips out and bake for around 25 minutes.

While the chips are cooking, get a large frying pan and heat the olive oil on a medium heat.

Pepper the steaks and add to the pan. Fry the steaks for 6 minutes in total, turning the steaks once halfway through.

Take the steak and leave to cool.

Get a large bowl and add the salad and chopped onion. Drizzle with the vinegar and serve with the potatoes and steak.

ORIENTAL
BEEF MUSCLE STIR-FRY

Great beef recipe, packed with loads of protein to keep you growing and burning fat.

CALORIES PER SERVING: 349

PROTEIN: 34G

CARBS: 26G

FAT: 14G

SERVES 4

500g of diced beef rump,

1 tsp Chinese five-spice powder

300g of egg noodles

1 large chopped red chilli

1 chopped garlic clove

1 chopped ginger

1 stick lemongrass

2 tbsp of olive oil

100g sugar snap peas

8 baby corn, sliced diagonally

6 chopped spring onions

½ lime

2 tbsp soy sauce

1 tbsp fish sauce

2 tbsp roasted peanuts

1 chopped coriander, to serve

HOW TO MAKE:

Get a bowl and add the beef and five-spice and leave to marinade. Place the egg noodles in a pot of boiling water for about 5 minutes, drain and then place to one side.

Mix together the chopped chilli, ginger, garlic and lemongrass in a bowl.

Add 1 tbsp of olive oil to a wok and heat on a medium heat. Add the ginger mixture into the wok and fry for 1 minute. Turn up the heat and add 1 more tbsp of olive oil to the wok and add the beef and fry until browned.

Add the sugar snaps, spring onions and baby corn to the wok and continue to stir-fry for around a minute before adding the egg noodles and mix together. Turn off the heat and add the soy sauce, fish sauces and squeezed lime juice.

Place in a bowl and add the peanuts and chopped coriander to serve.

BRAWNY BEEF FAJITAS

Quick and easy beef recipe, perfect for lunch, packed with loads of protein to keep you growing and burning fat.

CALORIES PER SERVING: 358

PROTEIN: 28G

CARBS: 40G

FAT: 10G

HOW TO MAKE:

Add the diced steak, chopped onion, red pepper and 1 tbsp of chilli sauce to a pan and stir fry for around 4 – 5 minutes.

Place the wrap in the microwave for 30 seconds

Add the steak mix to the fajita and along with one more tbsp of sweet chilli sauce, roll up and enjoy

SERVES 1

100g of diced lean steak

1 chopped red onion

1 chopped red pepper

1 wholegrain fajita wrap

2 tbsp of sweet chilli sauce

BULK-UP
LAMB CURRY & PEANUT STEW

This absolutely delicious curry is packed full of flavour and has a hefty does of protein to boot.

CALORIES PER SERVING: 600

PROTEIN: 44G

CARBS: 38G

FAT: 46G

SERVES 4

50g chopped peanuts

400ml can coconut cream

4 tbsp massaman curry paste

600g diced lamb steak (or beef)

450g chopped white potatoes

1 chopped onion

1 cinnamon stick

1 tbsp tamarind paste

1 tbsp fish sauce

1 sliced red chilli

HOW TO MAKE:

Pre-heat oven (375°F/190 °C/Gas Mark 5).

Get a large casserole dish and place on the gas/electric hob on a medium heat.

Add 2 tbsp of coconut cream and the curry paste and fry for around a minute before adding the diced lamb. Stir in and brown. Add the rest of the coconut cream with a cup of water as well as the potatoes, onions, cinnamon stick, tamarind, fish sauce and peanuts.

Reduce heat to a simmer, cover the casserole, transfer to the oven and cook for 2 hours until the lamb is soft and tender.

Add the sliced chilli to the top and serve.

MIGHTY
LAMB CASSEROLE

This absolutely delicious curry is packed full of flavour and has a hefty does of protein to boot.

CALORIES PER SERVING: 380

PROTEIN: 35G

CARBS: 33G

FAT: 9G

SERVES 2

1 tbsp of olive oil

2 cubed lamb fillets

1 chopped onion,

2 chopped carrots, thickly sliced

Handful of kale

400ml of chicken stock

1 tsp dried rosemary

1 tsp of chopped parsley

400g of rinsed and drained
cannellini beans

HOW TO MAKE:

Get a large casserole dish and heat the olive oil on a medium heat.

Add the lamb to the casserole dish and cook for 5 minutes until browned, then add the chopped onion and carrots. Leave to cook for another 5 minutes until the vegetables begin to soften.

Add the chicken stock, kale and rosemary. Then cover the casserole, leave to simmer on a low heat for 1-1.5 hours until the lamb is tender and fully cooked through.

Add the cannellini beans 15 minutes before the end of the cooking time.

Plate up and serve with the chopped parsley to garnish.

STEAK & CHEESE MUSCLE CLUB

A very quick and easy, tasty, healthy homemade sandwich with a generous amount of protein to ensure you continue to build muscle and burn fat.

CALORIES PER SERVING: 336

PROTEIN: 32G

CARBS: 27G

FAT: 11G

SERVES 2

1 250g sirloin steak

2 whole-meal bread rolls

1 tsp olive oil

1 tsp Dijon mustard

Handful of rocket

30g Stilton cheese

1 tsp of balsamic vinegar

A pinch of salt and pepper

HOW TO MAKE:

Heat up a griddle pan on a high heat until very hot. Drizzle the olive oil over the steak over both sides of the steak. Sprinkle some salt and pepper over it and place the steak in the pan and fry for 3 minutes on each side.

Place the steak to one side and leave to rest for a minute.

Cut in half to form two slices of steak.

Cut the whole-wheat rolls in half and place toast. Once done, add the mustard and rocket to the roll and place 1 half of the steak on top. Add balsamic vinegar and the cheese to the top and then make the sandwich.

Repeat steps with the other roll.

MASS GAINING LAMB FLATBREAD

A tasty and healthy homemade flatbread with a Moroccan twist, including a generous amount of protein to fuel you and your muscles!

CALORIES PER SERVING: 391

PROTEIN: 29G

CARBS: 34G

FAT: 17G

SERVES 4

2 200g lamb leg steaks

1 tbsp harissa

4 whole meal flatbreads

4 tbsp of organic houmous

Handful of baby spinach

Handful of watercress

A pinch of salt and pepper

HOW TO MAKE:

Preheat the grill.

Sprinkle harissa, salt and pepper over the lamb.

Place lamb on a baking tray and grill for 4 minutes before turning the lamb over and cooking for a further 4 minutes. Take the tray out of the grill and leave to one side.

Place the flatbreads under the grill for around 1 – 2 minutes before removing and spreading on the houmous.

Cut the lamb into thin strips and place over the flat bread.

Add the baby spinach and watercress, roll the flatbread into a wrap and enjoy.

SUPER STEAK, SPICY RICE & BEANS

The perfect steak...

CALORIES PER SERVING: 650

PROTEIN: 48G

CARBS: 60G

FAT: 26G

SERVES 2

2 250g sirloin steaks

4 tsp olive oil

1 small onion, sliced

100g brown long-grain rice

1½tsp fajita seasoning

1 can of drained kidney beans

Handful of chopped coriander leaves

2 tbsp tomato salsa, to serve

HOW TO MAKE:

Pour 3 tsp of oil into a deep saucepan on a medium heat and add the onion. Fry the onion for around 4 minutes.

Then add ½ the fajita seasoning and long grain rice. Cook for 1 minute. Add 300ml of boiling water to the saucepan and stir in. Cover the saucepan and let simmer for 20 minutes until the water has been absorbed and the rice is fluffy. Add the kidney beans and keep the pan warm.

While the rice is cooking, sprinkle salt and pepper over the steak as well as ½ fajita seasoning. Pre-heat a griddle pan on a high heat, add the steaks and cook for 8 minutes in total, turning the steaks half way through.

Add the rice to a bowl and mix in the coriander. Add a tbsp of tomato salsa to each of the steaks and serve.

MUSCLE
MINT LAMB STEAKS

Delicious recipe with over 40g of protein to keep you building muscle and burning fat.

CALORIES PER SERVING: 367

PROTEIN: 41G

CARBS: 2G

FAT: 22G

HOW TO MAKE:

Get a bowl and add the mint, vinegar and garlic and mix together.

Add the lamb to the bowl and leave to marinade for at least 30 minutes.

Pre-heat a griddle pan on a medium to high heat and cook the lamb for 4 minutes each side or until cooked through.

Serve alone or with your choice of salad for a delicious accompaniment.

SERVES 2

4 200g lamb leg steaks

2 tbsp olive oil

2 chopped garlic cloves

1 tbsp balsamic vinegar

Handful of chopped mint leaves

SUPER
LAMB STEAKS WITH MEDITERRANEAN VEG

A mediterranean twist on a lamb dish! A very quick and easy, healthy lamb recipe to keep you going for longer...

CALORIES PER SERVING: 308

PROTEIN: 34G

CARBS: 15G

FAT: 14G

HOW TO MAKE:

Add the oil to a pan and heat. Throw in the courgettes, tomatoes and garlic and fry until courgettes and tomatoes are soft. Add the rocket and coriander and stir in.

Meanwhile, sprinkle some salt and pepper over the lamb steaks. Place the lamb on a tray and grill for 4 minutes each side. Serve with the veg.

SERVES 2

2 lamb leg steaks

2 chopped courgettes

2 tbsp olive oil

Handful of rocket

2 garlic cloves, chopped

8 halved baby cherry tomatoes,

Handful of chopped coriander

STRENGTH AND MASS MEATLOAF

The perfect muscle building meatloaf!

CALORIES PER SERVING: 410

PROTEIN: 47G

CARBS: 15G

FAT: 19G

SERVES 6

900g of lean ground beef

1 tsp olive oil

1 chopped red onion

1 tsp garlic

3 chopped tomatoes

1 whole beaten egg

100g of whole wheat bread crumbs

Handful of parsley

20g of low fat parmesan

50ml of organic skim milk

A pinch of salt and pepper

1 tsp oregano

HOW TO MAKE:

Preheat the oven to (400°F/200 °C/Gas Mark 6).

Add the oil to a pan and heat on a medium heat.

Cook the onions until soft but not browned. Remove the onions from the pan and let cool.

Get a big bowl and mix all of the ingredients together.

Put the meat in a big baking tray and cook on a high heat for around 30-35 minutes.

Serve once cooked through and piping hot.

FARLEY'S
MUSCLE BUILDING CHILLI CON CARNE

Who doesn't like Chilli con carne? Well this healthy version will provide you with over 30g of protein and a smug sense of satisfaction!

CALORIES PER SERVING: 389

PROTEIN: 37G

CARBS: 25G

FAT: 17G

SERVES 4

500g lean ground beef	400g of tinned chopped tomatoes
1 tbsp oil	
	2 tbsp tomato purée
1 chopped onion	
1 chopped red pepper	400g of dried and rinsed red kidney beans
2 crushed garlic cloves,	
	100g of brown rice
1 tsp of chilli powder	
1 tsp paprika	
1 tsp ground cumin	
1 beef stock cube	

HOW TO MAKE:

Get a pan and add the olive oil and heat on a medium heat.

Add the onions to the pan and fry until soft.

Then add the garlic, red pepper, chilli powder, paprika and cumin. Stir together and cook for 5 minutes.

Add the ground mince to the pan and cook until browned.

Get 300ml of hot water and add the beef stock cube to it. Add this to the pan along with the chopped tomatoes. Also add the puree and stir in well. Bring the pan to a simmer, cover and cook for around 50 minutes. Stir occasionally.

After 30 minutes and while the mince is cooking, add 300ml of cold water to a separate pot and heat until the water is boiling. Once boiling, add the rice and leave for 20 minutes.

Once the rice is done, drain and put to one side. Add the beans to the meat mix and cook for another 10 minutes.

Serve the rice topped with the chilli con carne.

TASTY
BEEF BROCCOLI STIR-FRY

A very quick and easy, healthy beef stir-fry that will save you reaching out for the local Chinese delivery menu!

CALORIES PER SERVING: 277

PROTEIN: 30G

CARBS: 7G

FAT: 14G

SERVES 4

400g of diced frying beef steaks

1 head of broccoli, broken into florets

4 chopped celery sticks

Handful of sweet corn

150ml beef stock

2 tbsp of horseradish sauce

1 tbsp of olive oil

A pinch of salt and pepper

HOW TO MAKE:

Heat the olive oil on a medium/high heat in a frying pan.

Add some salt and pepper to the beefsteaks and place in the frying pan.

Stir-fry for 2 minutes until the beef is browned then remove and set aside.

Add the broccoli and chopped celery to the pan and fry for a further 2 minutes.

Add the beef stock to the pan, then cover. Reduce the heat and let the veg simmer for 2 minutes.

Place the steak back in the pan and mix with the other vegetables for another minute.

Plate up and serve with the horseradish sauce.

FISH AND SEAFOOD

A lot of us reserve fish for the refined. Either that or we're scared of cooking it. Fish is often easier than cooking meat; it's fresh, healthy and full of omega 3. Hopefully the recipes provided in this section will either get you started with cooking up fish, or further you down the chef road you're already on. Oh, and it will mean you burn fat, build strength, and increase brain power all at the same time!

MUSCLE
MACKEREL AND SPICY COUSCOUS

Mackerel is a great healthy source of protein and is also a great source of omega-3 fats.

CALORIES PER SERVING: 484

PROTEIN: 26G

CARBS: 35G

FAT: 26G

SERVES 1

150g of couscous

100g of pre cooked mackerel

1tsp of ground cumin

1 tsp of smoked paprika

1 chopped red chilli

Pinch of black pepper

2 chopped tomatoes

1 chopped onion

Handful of chopped mint

HOW TO MAKE:

Pour the couscous into a bowl and add the cumin, smoked paprika and pinch of black pepper. Then grab a cup of boiling water and pour it over the couscous until it covers it by about 1cm. Cover the bowl and leave for around 10-15 minutes.

When the water has been absorbed, add the chopped chilli, chopped tomatoes, chopped mint and chopped onion to the bowl and stir.

Add the mackerel to the top and serve.

SUPER COD
AND VEG

A simple recipe that's quick and easy to make and tasty too. You guessed it - high in protein and low in carbs!

CALORIES PER SERVING: 324

PROTEIN: 28G

CARBS: 11G

FAT: 19G

SERVES 1

140g fillet of white fish (Boneless)

1 cup of frozen peas

Salt

Pepper

1 tbsp of olive oil

2 sliced spring onions

1 chopped gem of lettuce

1 tbsp reduced-fat crème fraîche

HOW TO MAKE:

Add the lettuce, spring onions, frozen peas and olive oil to a microwave-proof bowl.

Season the fish with salt and pepper and 1 tbsp crème fraîche and add to the bowl.

Cover the bowl with cling film; pierce it several times with a fork and place in microwave.

Microwave the bowl for around 8 minutes until the fish as been fully cooked and is piping hot throughout.

Take the bowl from the microwave and remove the fish, placing to one side.

Use a fork to mash the vegetables and serve topped with the fish and an extra spoonful of crème fraîche.

LEMONY SALMON

Salmon is a great source of protein and is very high in omega 3 fats. Most salmon dishes can be bland and boring...Not this one!

CALORIES PER SERVING: 205

PROTEIN: 20G

CARBS: 1G

FAT: 13G

SERVES 4

4 100g Salmon fillets

1 lemon

A pinch of salt and pepper

10g of chopped tarragon

Handful of rocket

2 tbsp of olive oil

1 chopped garlic clove

HOW TO MAKE:

Pre-Heat grill.

Get a bowl and add the chopped garlic, tarragon, sprinkle of salt, sprinkle of pepper and olive oil. Squeeze the lemon juice and zest in the bowl and mix everything together.

Add the salmon fillets to the bowl and coat them in the marinade. Cover the bowl and leave the salmon fillets to marinade for 10 minutes.

Take the salmon fillets out of the bowl and place on a tray, pouring the marinade over the top of the fillets.

Grill the salmon fillets for around 10 minutes or until cooked through.

Plate up and serve.

STRENGTHENING SUB-CONTINENTAL SARDINES

Sardines are a great source of protein as well as omega 3's.

CALORIES PER SERVING: 356

PROTEIN: 20G

CARBS: 52G

FAT: 7G

SERVES 4

50g plain flour

10 sardines, scaled and cleaned (8 if large)

Zest 2 lemons

Large bunch of chopped flat-leaf parsley,

3 garlic cloves, finely chopped

3 tbsp olive oil

400g of tinned chopped tomatoes

800g chickpeas or butterbeans, drained and rinsed

250g pack cherry tomatoes, halved

A pinch of salt and pepper

HOW TO MAKE:

Sprinkle the flour with salt and pepper and spread the flour out on the work surface.

Cover the sardines with the flour on each side.

Now in a separate bowl add the lemon zest to the chopped parsley (save a pinch for garnishing) and half of the chopped garlic, ready for later.

Put a very large pan on the grill and heat on high.

Now add the oil and once very hot, lay the floured sardines flat.

Fry for 3 minutes until golden underneath and turn over to fry for another 3 minutes. Put these onto a plate to rest.

Fry the remaining garlic (add another splash of oil if you need to) for 1 min until softened. Pour in the tin of chopped tomatoes, mix and let simmer for 4-5 minutes.

Tip in the chickpeas or butter beans and fresh tomatoes, then stir until heated through.

Here's when you add the sardines into the lemon and parsley mix and cook for a further 3-4 minutes.

Once they're cooked through, serve with a pinch of parsley to garnish.

MUSCLE BUILDING SARDINES ON TOAST

A quick and easy muscle-building recipe to make: perfect for lunches or snacks.

CALORIES PER SERVING: 442

PROTEIN: 24G

CARBS: 30G

FAT: 23G

SERVES 2

4 slices Ezekiel bread or whole wheat brown bread

2 cans of drained sardines in olive oil

1 tbsp olive oil

1 chopped garlic clove

1 chopped red chilli

1 lemon, zest and juice

Small bunch of chopped parsley

HOW TO MAKE:

Toast the bread.

Heat some olive oil in a pan on a medium heat.

Add the chilli, garlic, lemon zest and sardines and heat for 2-3 minutes until cooked.

Place the sardines on the toast and sprinkle the parsley over them. Finish off with a few drops of lemon juice to serve.

MIGHTY TUNA MELTS

Not sure what to do with that tuna can at the back of the cupboard? This is a delicious protein pack recipe that's ready in minutes..

CALORIES PER SERVING: 450

PROTEIN: 37G

CARBS: 20G

FAT: 24G

SERVES 4

200g of tinned, drained tuna

Handful of chopped spring onions

4 tbsp low-fat mayonnaise

4 thick slices wholemeal bread

50g grated cheddar

2 tbsp of chilli flakes

1 squeezed lemon

A pinch of salt and pepper

HOW TO MAKE:

Toast the bread and pre-heat the grill.

Get a bowl and add the spring onions, mayonnaise, tuna and chilli flakes along with salt and pepper and the lemon juice. Mix everything together.

Spread the tuna mix over the top of the slices of bread and sprinkle the grated cheese over the top. Place under the grill until the cheese starts to bubble.

Plate up and serve.

TASTY TUNA,
BROCCOLI & CAULIFLOWER PASTA BAKE

Delicious pasta meal packed with protein for all your muscle-building and fat loss needs.

CALORIES PER SERVING: 641

PROTEIN: 37G

CARBS: 73G

FAT: 22G

SERVES 4

2 cans of tuna in olive oil (drained)

800g of canned chopped tomatoes

350g whole-wheat pasta

150g chopped broccoli

150g chopped cauliflower

200g pack light soft cheese

100g of grated cheddar

25g whole-wheat breadcrumbs

1 tbsp of Olive oil

HOW TO MAKE:

Grab a pan and heat the olive oil (medium/high heat).

Add the canned tomatoes and 200ml of water and let simmer.

Heat another large pan of water until it boils. Add the whole-wheat pasta and leave until the pan starts to boil again. Reduce the heat until the water simmers. Leave the whole-wheat pasta to cook for around 10 minutes. Add the broccoli and cauliflower during the last 3 minutes then drain.

Whilst the pasta and veg is cooking, pre heat the grill.

Add the cheese to the tomato sauce and stir until it melts, then add the drained pasta, vegetables and tuna.

Pour the mixture in a deep tray and cover with the cheddar, breadcrumbs, salt and pepper.

Place under the grill and cook for 6 minutes until golden.

Plate up and serve.

SUPERHUMAN
SEA BASS WITH SIZZLING SPICES

A delicious meaty meal that's packed full of protein.

CALORIES PER SERVING: 202

PROTEIN: 28G

CARBS: 2G

FAT: 9G

SERVES 6

6 x sea bass fillets skin on and scaled

3 tbsp olive oil

1 thumb-size piece of ginger, peeled and chopped into slices

3 thinly sliced garlic cloves

3 red chillies deseeded and thinly sliced

5 sliced spring onion stems

1 tbsp soy sauce

HOW TO MAKE:

Get a large pan and heat 2 tbsp of the oil on a medium heat.

Sprinkle salt and pepper over the Sea Bass and score the skin of the fish a few times with a sharp knife.

Add the sea bass fillet to the very hot pan with the skin side down (you must press the fish down onto the pan with your cooking spatula to prevent the fish from shrivelling and shrinking).

Cook the fish this way for around 5 minutes, or until you can see the skin underneath turning golden brown (you can lose the pressure on the spatula after the first few seconds)!

Now turn the fish over for around 30 seconds to give the flesh a nice golden colour.

Take the fish out of the pan, and place to one side.

Add the rest of the oil to the pan, throw in the chillies, garlic and ginger and cook for approximately 2 minutes or until golden.

Take this off the heat and add the spring onions with the soy sauce. Pour the sauce over your sea bass for a delicious oriental treat.

PROTEIN PACKED PAELLA

A delicious, traditional Spanish dish that's packed full over flavour and protein to ensure you continue to build muscle and burn fat.

CALORIES PER SERVING: 351

PROTEIN: 21G

CARBS: 50G

FAT: 9G

HOW TO MAKE:

Heat olive oil in a pan on a high heat. Add the chorizo, onion and garlic and then fry for 2-3 minutes until soft.

Add the turmeric, rice, prawns and frozen peas as well as 100ml of boiling water.

Stir until everything is warm and the water has been absorbed.

Plate up and serve.

SERVES 4

200g frozen cooked prawns

2 diced chorizo sausages

1 tbsp olive oil

1 chopped onion

1 chopped garlic clove

½ tsp turmeric

600g cooked brown rice

100g frozen peas

BRAWNY BAKED
HADDOCK WITH SPINACH AND PEA RISOTTO

Haddock is cheap and easy to cook and on top of this is packed full of nutrients and is a warm and wholesome filler!

CALORIES PER SERVING: 469

PROTEIN: 32G

CARBS: 66G

FAT: 10G

SERVES 4

400g skinless, boneless, smoked haddock from your local fishmonger or supermarket

1 tbsp olive oil

1 onion, chopped

300g risotto rice

450ml of vegetable stock

250g fresh spinach leaves

Handful of frozen peas

3 tbsp crème fraîche

50g grated parmesan cheese

A pinch of pepper

HOW TO MAKE:

Heat the oil in a large pan or wok on a medium heat.

Fry the chopped onion until just soft (not brown) before adding in the rice and stirring until soft.

Now add half of the stock and continue to stir slowly until the rice takes on a translucent texture.

Keep adding the rest of the stock slowly whilst stirring for up to 20-30 minutes.

Stir in the spinach and peas to the risotto.

Place the fish on top of the rice, replace the lid, then let steam for 10 minutes.

Flake the fish into large chunks and stir into the rice with the crème fraîche and half the parmesan.

Sprinkle with freshly ground pepper, then add the rest of the parmesan on top to taste!

RUSTIC
SCALLOPS WITH CORIANDER AND LIME

Scallops are a delicacy and if you feel like pushing the boat out, a great tasty change from the norm!

CALORIES PER SERVING: 225

PROTEIN: 20G

CARBS: 3G

FAT: 14G

HOW TO MAKE:

Heat pan on a medium to high and fry scallops for about 1 minute each side until golden. Add the chopped chilli and garlic cloves to the pan and squeeze the lime juice over the scallops.

Remove the scallops and sprinkle the chilli and coriander over them as well as some salt and pepper to serve.

SERVES 4

8 queen or king scallops (row on)

1 tbsp olive oil

2 large chopped garlic cloves

1 tsp chopped fresh red chilli

1/2 lime juice

2 tbsp of chopped coriander

A pinch of salt and pepper

TRAINING
TILAPIA IN THAI SAUCE

Tilapia is an exotic sounding fish but can often be found in your local fishmonger or superstore counter. Failing this, you can use this recipe with Sea bass or any other fish fillets of your choice!

CALORIES PER SERVING: 328

PROTEIN: 28G

CARBS: 25G

FAT: 14G

SERVES 4

4 tilapia fillets

2 tbsp flour

2 tbsp olive oil

4 spring onions, sliced

1 stick of chopped lemon grass

2 crushed garlic cloves

Small piece of chopped fresh ginger

2 tbsp soy sauce

Lime juice 1 lime, plus 1 lime chopped into wedges, to serve

1 chopped red chilli

Handful of coriander leaves

HOW TO MAKE:

Dip the tilapia fillets into the flour so that the whole fillet is coated.

Add olive oil to a pan on a medium to high heat and fry the fillets for 3 minutes on each side.

Using the same pan, fry the garlic, chilli, lemon grass and ginger on a low heat, adding the soy sauce and lime juice and simmering until the sauce thickens slightly.

Spoon the sauce over the fish and add the spring onions for a couple of minutes before dishing up and garnishing with your choice of herb and the lime wedges on the side.

TANGY TROUT

Trout is the king of all river fish and its goodness cannot be underrated! Sea trout is just as majestic so don't rule it out!

CALORIES PER SERVING: 298

PROTEIN: 30G

CARBS: 10G

FAT: 16G

SERVES 4

4 trout fillets

50g whole wheat/brown breadcrumbs (you can buy these pre-packaged or just use your trusty blender to wiz up your crust ends!)

1 tbsp olive oil

1 small chopped bunch parsley

Zest and juice of 1 lemon

25g toasted and chopped pine nuts or walnuts

HOW TO MAKE:

Turn your grill up high.

In the meantime, spread a little oil over a baking tray and mix the breadcrumbs, parsley, lemon zest and juice and half of the nuts.

Lay the fillets skin side down onto your tray and rub into your mixture on both sides before drizzling with more olive oil.

Leave them under the grill for five minutes and then scatter over the rest of the nuts to serve.

STEAMY WORKOUT FISH

This dish is fresh and delicious; it's so easy to cook and you can pack it full with extra greens and vitamins!

CALORIES PER SERVING: 145

PROTEIN: 29G

CARBS: 4G

FAT: 1G

SERVES 4

Tin foil, greaseproof paper or baking paper.

100g pak choi

4 x 150g fillets firm white fish (Cod, Plaice, Pollock, Seabass or Haddock)

2 garlic cloves, finely chopped

2 tbsp soy sauce

1 tsp mirin rice wine

4 chopped spring onions stems

HOW TO MAKE:

Heat oven to (200°C/400°F/Gas Mark 6).

You're going to be making a parcel for your delicious ingredients so you will need tin foil, greaseproof paper or baking paper.

Cut off four large rectangles and place each fillet on each piece of paper.

Add the garlic, soy sauce and rice wine.

You may want to use one or two of the lime wedges to squeeze the juices into your parcel.

Fold these up into a parcel leaving one edge open.

Cook for 20 minutes then add the spring onions and chilli for a fresh taste to end.

JOCK'S
JACKET POTATO WITH TUNA

Who said a jacket potato had to be boring? Try this sweet potato version and you'll be left satisfied and full with your fair share of protein!

CALORIES PER SERVING: 352

PROTEIN: 33G

CARBS: 27G

FAT: 13G

SERVES 1

1 large sweet potato

185g can tuna in olive oil, drained

½ finely chopped red onion,

1 small deseeded and chopped red chilli, (dried chilli will be just as good)

1 tbsp natural yoghurt

A bunch of chopped spring onions

HOW TO MAKE:

Preheat the oven to (200°C/400°F/Gas Mark 6).

You don't need to peel the sweet potato but you may want to scrape off the nobly bits with a sharp knife!

Pierce the potato with a fork multiple times and place in the microwave for 20 minutes (if you don't have a microwave you can use the oven but it will take around 30 minutes).

Whilst it's cooking, mix the tuna with the chopped onion and chill and season with salt and pepper.

Place the sweet potato in the pre-heated oven for a further 5-10 minutes or until a little crispy and serve with the tuna mix and yoghurt over the top.

Sprinkle the chopped spring onion over that!

SALADS

Salads are boring right? They're only designed for rabbits and skinny women on diets. Wrong. Salads done right are firstly delicious and don't have to just be a side; secondly they can be stuffed with fibre, protein, vitamins, nutrients. Don't make the stupid error of ignoring our trusted training companions and try a salad soon.

TUNA, SPINACH & QUINOA SALAD

Quick and easy tasty tuna salad for your muscle building and fat loss needs.

CALORIES PER SERVING: 302

PROTEIN: 18G

CARBS: 28G

FAT: 13G

SERVES 2

2 cans of tinned tuna in olive oil

Handful of baby spinach

1 chopped red onion

300g of chopped peppers

1 tbsp olive oil

1 chopped red chilli

225g of quinoa

350g of halved cherry tomatoes

1 cup of chopped black olives

HOW TO MAKE:

Add the quinoa to a large pan of boiling water and cook for 10 – 15 minutes until tender, then drain.

Heat oil in a pan on a medium heat and fry the onions, peppers and chilli until softened.

Get a bowl and add the drained quinoa, onion mix, tomatoes, tuna, baby spinach and olives and mix together.

Serve and enjoy

MEDITERRANEAN
SUPER SALAD

Quinoa's goodness cannot be overstated, this salad is packed full of protein and is also delicious too.

CALORIES PER SERVING: 290

PROTEIN: 15G

CARBS: 35G

FAT: 10G

SERVES 1

200g quinoa

1 tsp olive oil

½ red onion, finely chopped

2 tbsp mint (fresh or dried) and roughly chopped

400g of Puy or red lentils rinsed and drained – you can buy the dried lentils but you need to leave them to soak over night.

¼ cucumber (skins off and diced)

100g crumbled feta cheese

Zest and juice of 1 orange

1 tbsp red or white wine vinegar

HOW TO MAKE:

Cook the quinoa in a large pan of boiling water for 10-15 minutes until soft, drain and set aside to cool.

Fry the onion in the oil over a medium heat.

Stir together with the quinoa, lentils, cucumber, feta, orange zest, chopped mint and juice and vinegar.

Best served chilled!

For the meat fans, cooked chicken or lamb would be a delicious addition to this dish!

HUNKED UP HALLOUMI

This cheese could almost be meat it's so chunky and filling!

SERVES 4

2 tbsp white wine vinegar

1 tsp olive oil

½ red onion thinly sliced

Handful of rocket leaves

½ juiced lemon

Handful of green/black olives

500g of sliced halloumi cheese

1 tbsp mayonnaise

½ chopped cucumber

A pinch of pepper

HOW TO MAKE:

Preheat the grill.

Lightly drizzle a baking tray with 1 tsp olive oil before grilling for 5 minutes, turning until browned and crisp on the edges.

Add the chopped olives, rocket, cucumber and red onion into a bowl and mix with 1 tsp olive oil and lemon juice.

Season with pepper and stir in the mayonnaise (optional).

Serve alone or with crusty brown pitta breads for an Aegean twist!

ROASTED BEETROOT, GOATS CHEESE & EGG SALAD

Whether you love it or hate it, beetroot is a super food containing nutrients you rarely find in your five portions a day! Give it a go if you never have, or try this take on it if you're already a fan.

CALORIES PER SERVING: 363

PROTEIN: 11G

CARBS: 18G

FAT: 28G

SERVES 1

200g cooked chopped beetroot (not in vinegar)

2 tbsp olive oil

Juice from 1 orange

2 eggs

1 tsp white wine vinegar

2 tbsp crème fraîche

1 tsp Dijon mustard

A few stalks of dill, finely chopped (fresh or dried)

70g of baby gem lettuce

Handful of walnuts

100g crumbled goats cheese

A pinch of salt and pepper

HOW TO MAKE:

Preheat oven to (200°C/400°F/Gas Mark 6).

Place the beetroot onto the lightly oiled baking tray with the juice from the orange, sprinkle with salt and pepper.

Roast for 20-25 minutes, turning them once whilst they're baking. If they start to dry out, add a little more olive oil.

Meanwhile, put the eggs in boiling water. Turn down the heat and simmer for 8 minutes (4 minutes if you like your yolks runny) then run under cold water to cool. Peel and halve.

Mix the remaining oil, crème fraîche, mustard, a tsp of white wine vinegar and chopped dill together. This is the dressing for your lettuce.

Serve the salad with the beetroot and goats cheese crumbled over the top and walnuts sprinkled throughout.

SPICY
MEXICAN BEAN STEW

This one is technically a salad but really it could pass on anyone's dinner table. You won't be left hungry after this one and you'll certainly feel the heat kick-starting your metabolism!

CALORIES PER SERVING: 395

PROTEIN: 20G

CARBS: 45G

FAT: 15G

SERVES 4

250g canned chick peas, drained

200g canned cannellini beans, drained

200g of tinned chopped tomatoes

2 tbsp olive oil

1 chopped red onion

190g of sliced chorizo

3 red chopped chillis

1 tbsp paprika

HOW TO MAKE:

Heat a large pan on a medium heat with 1 tbsp olive oil, and cook the onion and chorizo for 5 minutes until lightly golden.

Tip in the chickpeas with the cannellini beans and stir until heated through.

Add the tin of chopped tomatoes and paprika and cover to let simmer for 5-10 minutes.

Serve – recommended with crusty brown bread, couscous or brown rice for a winter warmer!

THE
SAILOR SALAD

Spinach was good enough for the well-known muscle-building sailor cartoon then and its more than good enough for you now; add a generous portion of the sailor's catch and you'll be growing bigger than he ever did.

CALORIES PER SERVING: 220

PROTEIN: 20G

CARBS: 12.5G

FAT: 10G

SERVES 4

2 cups of chopped spinach (fresh)*

170g of lean grilled chopped turkey breast (or turkey deli meat already cooked)

1tbsp real bacon bits (you can cut up bacon and grill this yourself or buy the pre-packaged stuff)

2 diced hard-boiled eggs

100g new/baby potatoes

1 deseeded and sliced red, yellow and green pepper

1 avocado peeled and sliced (do this near to the end or it will start to turn brown)

1 tbsp balsamic vinegar

HOW TO MAKE:

Boil a medium sized pan of water on a high heat and add the halved new potatoes, cooking for 15-20 minutes or according to packaging guidelines.

Combine the meats (once grilled and chopped if you're doing this yourself) with the spinach and peppers in a serving bowl.

Drain the potatoes and let cool whilst placing a small pan to boil for the eggs. Cook for 8 minutes for medium-boiled or 10 minutes for hard-boiled eggs.

Run the eggs under a cold tap and peel. Dice and add to your salad (here's where you can peel the avocado and add this).

Stir through with balsamic vinegar and salt and pepper to taste.

SIZZLING
SALMON SALAD

Some like it hot. You can serve this one up with warm or cold salmon – either way it's wholesome and mouth-watering.

CALORIES PER SERVING: 521

PROTEIN: 46G

CARBS: 24G

FAT: 27G

SERVES 1

150g fillet salmon

6 cherry tomatoes

100g of couscous

3 stems of asparagus (chop off the very end of the base but leave the rest intact)

50g of diced low-fat mozzarella cheese

1 bell pepper sliced

1 tbsp balsamic vinegar

1 tbsp olive oil

A pinch of salt and pepper

HOW TO MAKE:

Preheat the grill.

Layer the couscous with boiling water from the kettle (about 1cm over the top of the couscous, cover and leave to steam)

Grill salmon for 10-15 minutes or until cooked through. Place to one side.

Uncover the couscous and stir through with a fork to break up the grains.

Now just add your pepper, mozzarella and halved cherry tomatoes to the couscous.

You will need to grill your asparagus for 3-4 minutes, turning every so often until lightly browned around the surface.

Once the asparagus is ready, place it along with the salmon on the bed of couscous and drizzle with olive oil and balsamic vinegar.

Salt and pepper to taste.

HERBY
TUNA STEAK

Protein, protein, protein!

CALORIES PER SERVING: 578

PROTEIN: 35G

CARBS: 3G

FAT: 48G

SERVES 2

2x 200g dolphin-friendly yellow fin tuna steaks

1 tbsp olive oil

2 lemon wedges

2 handfuls of flat-leaf parsley and 2 handfuls of coriander very roughly chopped

2 cloves of finely chopped garlic

½ onion finely chopped

Handful chopped green olives

6 tbsp olive oil

50g pine nuts or walnuts

Juice of half a lemon

HOW TO MAKE:

Your first job is the herby salad – mix the herbs with half of the chopped garlic, lemon juice and olive oil.

Crush the nuts in a tea towel or blend them up in your blender. Stir them in to the herbs.

Brush the tuna steaks with olive oil and sprinkle with salt and pepper.

You need to heat dry pan to an extremely high heat (look out for the smoke)

Seal the tuna in the pan for one minute on each side (if you have a griddle pan or grill then you should place these against the lines to get that nice straight off the BBQ look and taste)

If you like your tuna less-pink cook for 2 minutes on each side for medium, 3 for medium well and 4 for well done (approximate times).

Once cooked serve straight away with your herby salad (pour this over as a dressing or on the side as an accompaniment)

MUSCLE BUILDING
STEAK & CHEESE SALAD

A very quick and easy, healthy muscle building salad.

SERVES 2

250 frying beef steak

1 chopped red onion

1 teaspoon of crushed garlic

Handful of baby spinach

Handful of watercress

Handful of lettuce

4 chopped baby tomatoes

2 tbsp of balsamic vinegar

1 tbsp olive oil

50g of blue cheese

A pinch of salt and pepper

HOW TO MAKE:

Sprinkle salt and pepper over the steak.

Add a tbsp of olive oil to a griddle pan on a high heat.

Place the steak in the pan and cook 8 minutes in total, turning the steak half way through. Take the steak off the pan and allow to cool.

Cut the steak into 2cm strips, then place back into the pan and cook for a further minute on a medium heat.

Get a bowl and add the chopped tomatoes, watercress, baby spinach, lettuce, garlic and onions. Place the steak strips in the bowl along with the vinegar and a tbsp of olive oil. Mix everything together and grate the blue cheese over the top.

ANABOLIC AVOCADO AND CHICKEN SALAD

A fresh and delicious salad, pleasing the meat eater and keeping you anabolic!

CALORIES PER SERVING: 389

PROTEIN: 36G

CARBS: 12G

FAT: 14G

HOW TO MAKE:

Heat some olive oil on a medium heat in a griddle pan.

Grill the chicken breast for about 10 minutes each side or until cooked through.

Cut the chicken breasts into chunks and serve with the watercress, spinach, rocket, tomato and sliced avocado.

Finish off the salad by drizzling over olive oil

SERVES 1

1 chicken breast

Handful of watercress

Handful of baby spinach

Handful of rocket

½ a sliced avocado

1 chopped Beef tomato

¼ sliced cucumber

2 tbsp of olive oil

STRENGTH
CHICKEN AND SESAME SALAD

Contains three sources of protein for all your muscle-building needs.

CALORIES PER SERVING: 430

PROTEIN: 20G

CARBS: 16G

FAT: 15G

SERVES 2

2 chicken breasts

3 tbsp of sesame oil

2 tsp of grated ginger

1 crushed garlic clove

1 chopped red chilli

1 diced red onion

Handful of basil leaves

Handful of coriander leaves

100g of baby spinach leaves

1 tsp of sesame seeds

4 chopped almonds

1 peeled and sliced mandarin

HOW TO MAKE:

Pre-heat the grill.

Add 2 tbsp sesame oil, chopped red chilli, crushed garlic and ginger into a bowl. Mix all the ingredients together.

Make a few deep cuts into the chicken breast and leave them to marinate in the mixture for roughly 3 hours.

Add the spinach leaves, coriander leaves, basil leaves, red onion, chopped almonds and sesame seeds to a bowl and mix together.

Remove the chicken and rub over the last of the marinade and grill for 10 minutes each side or until fully cooked.

Cut the chicken into strips and add to the salad bowl.

Add the mandarin to the bowl and drizzle 1 tbsp of sesame oil over the salad and serve.

SIDES

Not enough to fill you up? Craving your side order of fries? Eyes bigger than your belly? No sweat. Here's a sweet collection of side orders you can prepare in your own home – add calories, protein and a little extra something, whilst knowing you've made it in the healthy way.

SWEET
POTATO WEDGES

Quick and easy. You won't be the only one devouring these tasty wedges.

CALORIES PER SERVING: 207

PROTEIN: 3G

CARBS: 38G

FAT: 6G

SERVES 4

4 sweet potatoes, scrubbed and cut
into large wedges

2 tbsp olive oil

3-4 cloves of garlic

Handful of rosemary sprigs

HOW TO MAKE:

Pre-heat oven to (350°F/180 °C/Gas Mark 4).

Once you've scrubbed the skin of the sweet potatoes (don't remove it)
with a kitchen scourer or something rough to suffice, you should toss the
wedges in olive oil.

Spread these out on a baking tray, sprinkling the rosemary sprigs over the
wedges and adding the whole garlic cloves in their skin over and around
the wedges. Pop the whole lot into a pre-heated oven for 30-40 minutes or
until crispy.

HOT & SPICY BUTTERNUT SQUASH

Often ignored in our fruit and veg selection, squash is a winner! One squash will feed a family, and if you're dining solo, freeze and save for another day!

CALORIES PER SERVING: 227

PROTEIN: 1G

CARBS: 30G

FAT: 14G

SERVES 4

1 butternut squash

4 tbsp olive oil

4 tbsp pouring honey

1 seeded and finely chopped red scotch bonnet chilli,

HOW TO MAKE:

Preheat the oven to (200°C/400°F/gas 6).

Chop the top and the bottom from the butternut squash. Next you need to cut it in half lengthways. You should now be able to use a vegetable peeler to remove the skin but if that doesn't work, take a sharp knife and cut downwards.

Now, using a spoon hollow out the seeds from the base.

You're free to slice now into thick (1-2 cm) slices horizontally.

On a lightly oiled baking tray, spread the slices into one layer across.

Drizzle the honey generously over the slices and sprinkle the chopped chili liberally (or according to heat tolerance!)

Bake for 35-40 minutes or until crispy.

Any left overs can be placed into a sealable sandwich bag and frozen – simply reheat in the oven when ready.

FRUITY
NUTTY QUINOA

Don't know what to do with your quinoa? This dish is absolutely delicious and will go great with most main meals.

CALORIES PER SERVING: 328

PROTEIN: 10G

CARBS: 36G

FAT: 15G

HOW TO MAKE:

Add the quinoa to a large pan of boiling water and then let simmer for 10 – 15 minutes until tender, then drain.

Get a bowl and add the quinoa, apricots, herbs, lemon juice, zest and olive oil along with some salt and pepper and mix together.

Scatter the cashews over the top and serve.

SERVES 2

200g quinoa

6 dried apricots

Juice of 1 lemon

2 tbsp olive oil

A pinch of salt and pepper

Handful of chopped parsley and mint

50g cashew nuts

RICE &
PEAS

Transport yourself to the Caribbean with this easy to prepare side dish.

CALORIES PER SERVING: 430

PROTEIN: 20G

CARBS: 16G

FAT: 15G

SERVES 2

300g brown rice

75ml olive oil

200g dried kidney beans

1 tsp chilli powder

HOW TO MAKE:

Soak the kidney beans in water overnight (you can buy tinned and use immediately if you're in a rush but you won't get that authentic color or taste!)

Boil the liquid with the kidney beans in using a large saucepan on a high heat (add water if you need to).

Add the rice and cook for 30 minutes and then drain. Keep the rice in the pan, add the kidney beans and cover and steam for 4 minutes.

Sprinkle chilli powder over your rice and serve

MUSCLE RICE SALAD

Add variety to your standard brown rice with this delicious and nutritious side..

CALORIES PER SERVING: 454

PROTEIN: 11G

CARBS: 64G

FAT: 19G

HOW TO MAKE:

Add 300ml of cold water to a pot and heat on high until the water is boiling.

Once boiling, add the rice and leave for 20 minutes. Then drain.

Mix the rice with chopped red pepper, chopped cucumber, grated carrot, cherry tomatoes and drizzle with olive oil.

SERVES 2

100g of brown rice

1 deseeded and finely chopped red pepper,

½ cucumber, deseeded and finely chopped

1 large grated carrot

1 cup of chopped cherry tomatoes

2 tbsp olive oil

LEMON
& MOROCCAN MINT COUSCOUS

A fresh and zingy side dish that works well with fish, chicken, vegetables, even lamb and beef.

CALORIES PER SERVING: 367

PROTEIN: 6G

CARBS: 43G

FAT: 20G

SERVES 2

250g couscous

2 tbsp grated zest of a lemon and the lemon juice

20g pack fresh mint

4 tbsp toasted pine nuts

HOW TO MAKE:

In a serving bowl, pour boiling water over the dried couscous (it needs to cover the couscous with about a cm on the top) and cover the bowl with a plate to steam. You could add a chicken/vegetable stock cube to the boiling water for seasoning if you wish.

Once the couscous has steamed for a few minutes uncover it and use a fork to 'fluff up' the grains.

Add the lemon zest and juice, finely chopped mint and pine nuts.

Season to taste and add a little olive oil to serve.

MUSHROOM
RISOTTO

Another dish that works well on the side – try it with chicken breast. Works great as a post workout side!

CALORIES PER SERVING: 445

PROTEIN: 15G

CARBS: 63G

FAT: 17G

SERVES 2

50g dried porcini mushrooms

1 vegetable stock cube

2 tbsp olive oil

1 finely chopped onion,

2 g finely chopped Garlic cloves,

250g sliced and washed pack chestnut mushrooms,

300g risotto rice, such as arborio

1 x 175ml white wine

Handful tarragon leaves chopped

50g freshly grated parmesan or grana padano,

HOW TO MAKE:

Pour 1 litre of boiling water over the dried porcini mushrooms and leave to soak for 20 minutes, then drain into a separate bowl (keep the liquid at this point as you need to add to the risotto later).

Chop the mushrooms into slices.

Heat up the oil on a medium heat in a large frying pan and add the onions and garlic, frying for around 5 minutes until they get soft.

At this point you should add the dried and fresh chestnut mushrooms and stir for another 5 minutes until softened.

Add the rice, stirring for a minute or so before adding all of the wine.

Let it get to simmering point (bubbling), and add a quarter of the mushroom stock.

Simmer the rice, stirring often, until the rice has absorbed all the liquid.

Keep adding the stock, a quarter at a time, each time waiting for the rice to absorb the liquid.

A lot of stirring is required until the rice is soft! If the liquid runs out and the rice is still a little hard you can continue to add small amounts of water.

When soft, take the pan off the heat and add half the cheese and tarragon leaves. Cover the pan and let it steam for a few minutes.

Serve with the rest of the cheese and herbs!

SWEDE & CARROT MASH UP

Try this home comfort – it's exciting mash!

CALORIES PER SERVING: 132

PROTEIN: 2G

CARBS: 22G

FAT: 5G

HOW TO MAKE:

Put the carrots, swede and garlic in a large pan of salted water, bring to the boil, and cook for 12 minutes. Add the tarragon and olive oil and season with salt and pepper.

Drain and then mash. Stir in a dollop of crème fraîche before serving if you like!

SERVES 4

500g chopped carrots

500g chopped swede

3 chopped garlic cloves

Handful of finely chopped tarragon,

1 tbsp olive oil

A pinch of salt and pepper

MUSTARDY CAULIFLOWER CHEESE

Winter Warmer – eat alone or on the side.

CALORIES PER SERVING: 240

PROTEIN: 15G

CARBS: 14G

FAT: 12G

SERVES 2

1 cauliflower

2 tbsp wholegrain mustard

100g mature cheddar cheese

100ml low-fat crème fraiche

HOW TO MAKE:

Chop the cauliflower by cutting off the thickest part of the stem and pulling apart the florets.

In a mixing bowl, place the cauliflower, ¾ of the cheese, crème fraîche and mustard and toss.

Place in an oven dish and pop into a preheated oven (200°C/400°F/gas 6) for 30 minutes.

Add the remaining cheese on to the top of the dish and grill for 5-7 minutes until brown and bubbling on top.

PALEO RECIPES

A BODYBUILDER'S GUIDE TO PALEO

A Paleo diet is meant to represent what a 'Cave-Man' would have been able to get his hands on back in the day. If a caveman couldn't catch it, pick it, drink it or eat it, then it's off limits my friend.

WHY PALEO?

Many experts feel that your nutritional habits make up to 80% of the way your body looks. Or in other words, if you eat like crap, chances are that you look like crap. Paleo, underneath all the jargon and in bodybuilding terms, is essentially a very clean, healthy diet. It's very high in protein, which of course is great for building muscle. It includes lots of fruit and veg, full of essential vitamins and minerals. The carbs including in the diet are slow releasing, which means a steady flow of energy is released into your body throughout the day.

As you can see, a paleo diet is a great way to burn fat, build muscle and obtain that aesthetic physique you're after!

SO WHAT IS ALLOWED

Meat (Grass-fed) – Beef, Pork, Chicken etc.

Seafood – All types of sustainable fish

Free range eggs

Fresh vegetables – the more the better!

Fresh fruit

High quality whey protein supplement

(I'm sure a caveman didn't have access to protein powder, but I felt that this should be included mainly for convenience; it can be quite difficult to reach your protein requirements just eating real meat)

Healthy oils – coconut oil, olive oil, macadamia oil

Nuts

Tubers – Sweet potatoes, yams, butternut squash

SO WHAT'S NOT ALLOWED?

Legumes

(this includes peanuts)

Dairy

Processed meat

Processed foods

Refined sugars

Refined vegetable oils

Candy

WHAT DOES IT LOOK LIKE ON MY PLATE?

Aim to have a high quality protein source with every meal along with a healthy serving of fruits, greens & veg.

PALEO FOR MUSCLE

On a Paleo diet, you will still need to take in an excess of calories along with the right nutrients in order to grow muscle. If you don't eat enough, your body won't be able to fully repair the damage you cause by lifting weights, thus triggering you to plateau or even worse - lose muscle.

PALEO TO SHRED

To lose fat, you need to take in fewer calories than you expend. Again if you don't take in the right nutrients and foods, you will lose muscle. As all the meals included in this diet and cookbook are inherently healthy and contain a good amount of protein, paleo is an ideal diet for gaining muscle and shredding fat!

CALCULATING YOUR MACROS

This chapter will provide you with a clear understanding of how to break down your diet and what it should consist of, including protein, carbohydrates and fats. It is vital to balance your meals between these three food categories in order to continue growing muscle and losing fat. What do you need to know about each of the following?

WHAT IS PROTEIN?

Protein is used by your body for a number of processes, from enzyme and hormone production to ensuring that your immune system is working to its optimum level. The reason why protein is so important in a muscle-building diet is because protein is absolutely critical for muscle growth and repair. Working out and "tearing down muscle" increases your body's need and demand for protein; as you build muscle, the more protein your body will require to repair, grow and maintain it. If you don't supply your body with enough protein, it will take it from your muscles therefore causing muscle breakdown. Making sure you get enough protein is therefore of upmost importance in planning your diet along with your training schedule..

WHAT ARE CARBOHYDRATES?

Carbohydrates get converted into glucose and are then used by your body for energy. There are two types of carbohydrate - simple and complex. Simple carbohydrates are found in foods like fruit. Complex carbohydrates are foods like sweet potatoes and vegetables. Complex carbohydrates tend to be thought of as the better of the two in terms of your diet. The difference between these types of carbohydrates is how long it takes the body to convert them into glucose. Simple carbohydrates are converted by your body quickly making them great for a fast source of energy however there is usually a fast decline in energy levels after. It takes your body a lot longer to convert complex carbohydrates into glucose making them a much more sustainable source of energy. The reason so many people are afraid of carbohydrates is because whatever your body doesn't use gets moved into your fat stores. However, carbohydrates are not the enemy, they are vital for energy and therefore the success of your training.

WHAT ARE FATS?

Fats are essential for many of your bodily functions. They are needed for the production of many hormones in your body and they also help keep your brain and nervous system running optimally. They are also the most calorically dense out of the three macronutrients – every gram of fat contains 9 calories!
There are four types of fat: monounsaturated, polyunsaturated, saturated and trans-fatty acids. The only types you need to avoid are trans-fatty acids. These are fats that have been modified in a lab to ensure a longer shelf life. The reason you should avoid trans-fatty acids is that the body does not know what to do with them as they are artificially modified and so they can cause cell damage.

HOW MUCH DO YOU NEED OF EACH ON A PALEO DIET?

Well that depends on your goals!

TO BUILD MUSCLE, A GOOD PLACE TO START FROM IS:

Bodyweight (lbs) x 17 = Total calories needed to build muscle.

Protein: 40%
Daily Calories needed x 0.4
Answer x 4 = amount in grams
Carbohydrates: 30%
Daily Calories needed x 0.3
Answer x 4 = amount in grams
Fats: 30%
Daily Calories needed x 0.3
Answer x 9 = amount in grams

You want to be gaining about 0.5 – 1 pound a week. Any more than that and you will be gaining too much fat. If you find you aren't gaining weight, increase your calories by around 100-200 cals each week until you reach the sweet spot. Alternatively if you're gaining too much, then you want to reduce your calories by around 100 – 200 each week.

TO GET SHREDDED, A GOOD PLACE TO START FROM IS:

Bodyweight (lbs) x 12 = Total calories needed to burn fat.

Protein: 40%
Daily Calories needed x 0.4
Answer x 4 = amount in grams
Carbohydrates: 30%
Daily Calories needed x 0.3
Answer x 4 = amount in grams
Fats: 30%
Daily Calories needed x 0.3
Answer x 9 = amount in grams

You want to be losing about 1 – 2 pound a week. Any more than that and you risk losing that hard earned muscle. If you find you aren't losing weight, decrease your calories by around 100-200 cals each week until you reach the sweet spot. Alternatively if you're losing too much, then you want to increase your calories by around 100 – 200 each week.

BREAKFAST

Being Paleo doesn't mean you have to skimp on meals or starve yourself in any way. Breakfast is still probably the most important meal of the day, especially in preparation for all the heavy weights you'll be lifting later on! Choose any one of these to get you set for training heavy

THE CAVEMAN'S
RED PEPPER CHICKEN OMELETTE

Transporting you back to your primordial days, this protein packed breakfast just got a little more exciting!

CALORIES PER SERVING: 326

PROTEIN: 30G

CARBS: 6G

FAT: 20G

SERVES 2

4 eggs (free range)

1 cooked and cubed chicken breast (free range)

1 tsp of olive oil

1 diced red onion

1 medium sliced red pepper

5 chopped cherry tomatoes

5-6 sliced mushrooms

Sprinkle of salt and pepper

HOW TO MAKE:

Crack and whisk the eggs, seasoning with salt and pepper in a separate bowl.

Heat the oil in a saucepan on high (but don't let it sizzle) before adding all of the ingredients minus the eggs.

Stir every so often to prevent sticking for 5-6 minutes or until vegetables softened and cooked.

Pour the egg mix evenly over the cooked vegetables, forming a circle (use a pan just the right size if possible).

Cook the egg for a further 7-8 minutes, using your spatula to lift the edges. If it comes away easily then you can flip it over. You can use the spatula for this or some wrist action if you're a pro-flipper!

Cook for another 2-3 minutes on the other side.

Simply plate and serve with a side of leaves if you wish.

SUPER-STRENGTH SPINACH SCRAMBLE

Another egg based breakfast, this time with extra strength and power, designed to keep you fit and get you raring to go.

CALORIES PER SERVING: 327

PROTEIN: 40G

CARBS: 8G

FAT: 15G

SERVES 2

3 eggs (free range)

5 egg whites (free range)

Handful of baby spinach

Handful of curly kale (or any other kale you can get your hands on)

½ small chopped onion

1 tsp of nutmeg (grated fresh or dried)

Sprinkle of pepper

1 tsp of olive oil

HOW TO MAKE:

Add olive oil to a large pan and place over medium/high heat. Add the chopped onions and kale and cook until soft and smelling delicious!

Now add all of your eggs to the pan, mixing quickly until scrambled. After 3-4 minutes add the spinach and the nutmeg along with pepper.

Continue to cook until it is to your liking – some like it soft and fluffy; others a little well done.

Plate and serve.

WARRIOR
STEAK AND EGG SUPREME

Who says steak has to be for dinner? Meat is most definitely paleo-perfect. Serve with eggs for a protein packed breakfast.

CALORIES PER SERVING: 283

PROTEIN: 35G

CARBS: 2G

FAT: 15G

SERVES 2

150g of rump beef steak (grass fed)

1-2 eggs (free range)

1 large beef tomato (cut in 2)

1 large field mushroom

HOW TO MAKE:

Heat a griddle pan/grill on high until very hot before adding the steak.

Cook using the following approximate timings for each side:

- 2 minutes = rare
- 3-4 minutes = medium
- 5-6 minutes = well done

Whilst the steak is cooking, add the tomato and mushroom to the pan, turning once through cooking.

Remove the steak and vegetables from the pan once done and allow to rest.

Heat a tsp of olive oil in the same pan and crack your eggs in. Cook until golden brown on the edges (3-4 minutes for a runny yolk and add a couple of minutes for a hard yolk).

Plate up and serve.

ACTION
AVOCADO AND BRAWNY BACON BOOST

Lots of protein and quick and easy to make. .

CALORIES PER SERVING: 422

PROTEIN: 23G

CARBS: 15G

FAT: 30G

SERVES 1

1 diced sweet potato

4 turkey bacon rashers

1 tbsp of olive oil

1 tsp of thyme

1 chopped avocado

1 chopped red onion

100g chopped mushrooms

Sprinkle of black pepper

HOW TO MAKE:

Heat a large saucepan over a medium heat and then add olive oil.

Add sweet potato cubes stirring frequently until sweet potatoes are tender but firm (about 12-15 minutes).

Whilst cooking the sweet potato, add small amounts of water (a few drops) to the pan and cover for a few minutes at a time to speed along the sweet potatoes.

Add the thyme, onions, bacon and mushrooms to the pan and cook for 6-7 minutes or until softened and the bacon is cooked through.

Plate and serve - top with avocado before seasoning with black pepper to taste.

SHRIMPIN' DELICIOUS OMELLETE

Turn your omelette into something a little more exciting.

CALORIES PER SERVING: 337

PROTEIN: 27G

CARBS: 33G

FAT: 9G

SERVES 1

4 beaten eggs (free range)

1 tsp of coconut oil

Sprinkle of black pepper

1 chopped red chilli

200g of shrimp (frozen or fresh)

HOW TO MAKE:

Cook shrimp and chilli over a medium heat until they turn pink if raw (if already cooked then make sure you cook until heated through).

Cut the shrimp into bite-size pieces and put to the side.

Whisk eggs in a separate small bowl.

Heat a non-stick pan on a medium-high heat.

Add coconut oil when hot.

Add the eggs to the pan, tilt it for a circular shape or use a pan that is the same size as you want your omelette to be.

Leave to cook on a low to medium heat for 4-5 minutes.

When eggs are almost fully firm, add shrimp pieces onto one half of the egg.

Fold omelette in half and cook for a minute more.

Plate and serve with a sprinkle of black pepper.

CITRUS AND SUPER BERRY PROTEIN PANCAKES

If you thought sweet, delicious pancakes were off your menu forever, think again!

CALORIES PER SERVING: 398

PROTEIN: 20G

CARBS: 30G

FAT: 22G

SERVES 2

2 tsp coconut oil

3 tbsp coconut flour

75g of almond meal

¼ tsp gluten-free baking soda

⅓ cup raisins

4 eggs

2 chopped bananas

1 tsp of ginger

Handful of blueberries

Zest and juice of 1 lemon

HOW TO MAKE:

Add eggs, banana, ginger, lemon zest, and 1 tsp coconut oil to a blender. Process for 15-20 seconds, until smooth and fluffy. (An electric whisk will do the trick or try a manual whisk to start your workout early!)

Sieve in the coconut flour and almond meal and baking soda.

Blend or whisk again until smooth.

Heat up a large frying pan on a medium heat and add another tsp of coconut oil when hot.

This will serve 1-2 hungry bodybuilders so divide the mixture accordingly and pour into the pan into individual rounded pancakes (go easy at first and pour your mixture into little circles, keep pouring whilst tilting the pan until you have a pancake to your desired shape).

Don't worry if they don't look perfectly formed, you'll have chance to practice these when you realize how great they taste.

These will need cooking on a medium heat for 2 minutes on each side. If you have enough for more than one batch, keep the oven warm and stack your pancakes on a plate to wait.

Add a little more coconut oil for frying your next batch!

Add the raisins and blueberries and add the juice of the lemon used for the citrus twist.

Plate and serve.

SPICED
PUMPKIN PANCAKES

Pancakes for when you're not in the mood for something sweet. These are tasty, filling and better than your average fatty treat when training.

CALORIES PER SERVING: 505

PROTEIN: 30G

CARBS: 21G

FAT: 34G

SERVES 1

Flesh from 1/4 deseeded pumpkin

4 eggs (free range)

3 egg whites (free range)

Sprinkle of black pepper

¼ tsp gluten-free baking soda

2 tbsp coconut oil

1 tbsp good quality maple syrup (not the commercial stuff found in big supermarkets – try local shops/ farm shops to ensure you're sticking to paleo!)

1 handful pecan nuts

HOW TO MAKE:

In a blender or food processor, blend the pumpkin flesh together with some water to form a smooth pulp.

Now add the eggs, freshly ground pepper, 1 tbsp of coconut oil, and a tiny pinch of baking soda to the pumpkin mix and blend until smooth.

Heat a large pan on a medium heat with the other 1 tbsp of coconut oil.

Pour into the pan into individual rounded pancakes (go easy at first and pour your mixture into little circles, keep pouring whilst tilting the pan until you have a pancake to your desired shape).

Lift the mixture with a spatula and then flip. Cook for 3 minutes on either side.

Plate and serve with pecan nuts and maple syrup.

CHICKEN AND POULTRY

Catch it. Kill it. Eat it. Or if you can't do the first two, at least you can rest assured that a cave man would have been able to! Chicken and poultry is certainly paleo-friendly, packed with protein, and low in fat. It's also delicious and adaptable. It needn't be a boring dry chicken breast and brown rice, usually associated with bodybuilding meal plans. Use these recipes to transform your preconceptions about chicken!.

CHICKEN
WITH HOMEMADE CHIPOTLE SAUCE

Smoky and spicy greatness, helping you build muscle.

CALORIES PER SERVING: 585

PROTEIN: 55G

CARBS: 17G

FAT: 33G

SERVES 2

4 free range chicken thighs (grilled)

7-10 chipotle peppers (stems removed and cut lengthways)

350g organic tomatoes (skin removed and blended)

250ml of water or homemade chicken broth

2 tbsp apple cider vinegar

1 white onion (minced)

2 cloves garlic (minced)

2 tbsp organic honey

1/2 tsp sea salt

1/2 tsp cumin

1 tsp cinnamon

1 tsp paprika

HOW TO MAKE:

Simmer all ingredients except the peppers and chicken thighs in a pan for 30 minutes (you could double up the ingredients and freeze half for future dipping!)

Add the peppers and simmer for another 30 minutes without the lid on.

Pour the sauce over the grilled chicken thighs.

Plate up and serve.

ANABOLIC
JERK CHICKEN

Add a little spice to your life with this traditional Caribbean dish. Packed full of protein and slow releasing carbohydrates to keep to you growing.

CALORIES PER SERVING: 516

PROTEIN: 32G

CARBS: 76G

FAT: 33G

SERVES 1

100g of chicken thighs or breast	½ of dried thyme
½ tsp of ground allspice	1 chopped onion
½ tsp of black pepper	2 scotch bonnet chillies
½ tsp of nutmeg	1/2 chopped red pepper
½ tsp of cinnamon	1 tsp of olive oil
½ tsp of sage	
½ tsp of dried thyme	
1 clove of garlic	

HOW TO MAKE:

To make the jerk paste, add allspice, nutmeg, sage, cinnamon, dried thyme, red pepper, black pepper, onion, olive oil, garlic, chopped red pepper and scotch bonnet chillies to the blender and blend into a puree.

Rub the paste over the chicken breasts and leave them for at least an hour to marinate or preferably overnight if possible.

Preheat the grill on a medium heat when ready to cook.

Add the chicken breasts to the grill for roughly 10-12 minutes per side or until they are cooked through and piping hot.

Plate up and serve with a side salad of your choice. Try the salads section later in the book for inspiration!

GRILLED CHICKEN KEBABS

A power-protein snack for the paleo palette; contains a whopping 73 grams of protein!

CALORIES PER SERVING: 488

PROTEIN: 73G

CARBS: 10G

FAT: 17G

SERVES 1

2 chicken breasts (free range)

2 minced garlic cloves

1 chopped red chilli (deseeded)

2 tbsp of sesame oil

1 red onion, chopped into eight pieces

Sprinkle of salt and pepper

3 wooden skewers

HOW TO MAKE:

Chop the chicken breasts into chunky pieces using a sharp knife or scissors.

Mix the sesame oil with the minced garlic, chilli and salt and pepper (as desired).

Marinate the chicken in half the oil and leave for at least one hour - if possible leave to marinate overnight.

Keep the rest of the oil for brushing whilst cooking.

Heat the grill to a high heat and soak wooden skewers in water.

Take skewers from the water and pierce a chunk of chicken followed by a slice of red onion – repeat this until skewer is covered.

Grill for 15-20 minutes, using a brush to rub the remaining oil over the chicken every five minutes and turning throughout.

Check there is no pink inside the chicken when cut and that it is boiling hot before serving).

SUPER
STICKY CHICKEN CLUBS

Caveman friendly!

CALORIES PER SERVING: 404

PROTEIN: 47G

CARBS: 37G

FAT: 8G

SERVES 4

8 free range chicken drumsticks

1 tbsp organic honey

1 tbsp olive oil

2 Beef tomatoes (organic when possible)

1 tbsp Dijon mustard

HOW TO MAKE:

Using a sharp knife, score each of the drumsticks.

Mix together the honey, oil, and mustard.

Pour this mixture over the chicken and coat thoroughly.

Leave to marinate for 30 minutes at room temperature or overnight in the fridge.

Preheat oven to (200°C /400°f/Gas Mark 6).

Tip the chicken into a shallow roasting tray, add the quartered tomatoes and cook for 35 minutes, turning occasionally, until the chicken is tender and glistening with the marinade.

Plate up and serve.

PALEO CHICKEN MUSHROOM BRAWN BURGER

One healthy burger! It's quick and easy to make if you're low on time, containing a good helping of protein to keep you anabolic.

CALORIES PER SERVING: 458

PROTEIN: 50G

CARBS: 38G

FAT: 12G

SERVES 1

4 portabella mushrooms (without the stalks)

2 tbsp of coconut oil

2 eggs (free range)

2 chicken breasts (free range)

1 chopped beef tomato

Sprinkle of salt and pepper

½ chopped iceberg lettuce

HOW TO MAKE:

Preheat grill on high.

Season chicken breasts with salt and pepper.

Place chicken in grill and cook for 20 minutes, turning chicken over half way through. Make sure chicken is cooked right through.

Heat coconut oil in pan on a medium heat.

Add mushrooms and sauté for 5 minutes until mushrooms are tender.

Remove mushrooms and place to one side.

Add the egg to the pan and fry on a medium heat for 4-5 minutes.

Serve the chicken and eggs on top of the two mushroom caps topped again with the lettuce and chopped tomatoes.

Plate up and enjoy!

TANGY
ORANGE AND CHICKEN THIGHS

Mix things up with this tangy chicken recipe.

CALORIES PER SERVING: 555

PROTEIN: 32G

CARBS: 25G

FAT: 35G

SERVES 2

300g of chicken thighs (free range)

Sprinkle of pepper

Juice of 2 oranges

Juice of 1 lime

2 tbsp of crushed ginger

2 tbsp of olive oil

2 peeled and pieced oranges

2 chopped cloves of garlic

1 chopped green pepper

HOW TO MAKE:

Heat oil in a large pan over a medium heat.

Season chicken thighs with pepper and add to the frying pan to brown.

After the chicken starts to brown, add garlic to the pan and stir for 1 minute.

Add the orange juice, ginger, lime, and oranges to the pan and stir well.

Cover the pan and bring to a simmer.

Cook chicken for around 25-30 minutes or until chicken is cooked through.

Plate up and serve.

SWEET
HONEY CHICKEN

Add a little sweet and savoury kick to your favourite protein source.

CALORIES PER SERVING: 479

PROTEIN: 42G

CARBS: 17G

FAT: 27G

SERVES 2

6 chicken drumsticks (free range)

Sprinkle of salt and pepper

2 tbsp of sesame oil

1 diced red pepper

1 finely diced chilli

1 tbsp of organic honey

3 minced garlic cloves

HOW TO MAKE:

In a bowl, add the honey chilli, garlic, diced red pepper, sesame oil, salt and pepper.

Mix them together.

Pour half of the honey mixture over the chicken drumsticks.

Make sure that the drumsticks are covered evenly.

Leave the chicken mix to marinate for at least 3 hours or overnight if possible.

Preheat the grill to a medium heat when ready.

Line a baking tray with tin foil and spread the chicken out evenly.

Grill under a medium heat for 25-30 minutes.

Check chicken is cooked through and piping hot before serving.

Plate up and serve.

DOUBLE WHAMMY

Contains a double dose of protein to keep you building muscle and burning fat.

::

CALORIES PER SERVING: 190

PROTEIN: 34G

CARBS: 2G

FAT: 5G

::

SERVES 4

900g of chicken thighs (free range)

110g of turkey bacon (or pork if you can't find turkey)

250ml of homemade chicken stock (see following recipe)

HOW TO MAKE:

Cut the bacon into small squares.

On a medium heat, cook the bacon in a pan in a little olive oil (not too much as the bacon will produce its own fat).

Remove the bacon and set aside.

Now add the chicken into the same pan and brown on all sides.

Add your homemade chicken stock and bring to the boil before reducing heat, covering and allowing to simmer for 20-30 minutes.

Once the chicken is soft and cooked through, add the bacon back to the pan and stir through.

Best served with a hunky corn on the cob, olive oil, salt and pepper to taste.

Plate and serve.

HOMEMADE
PALEO CHICKEN STOCK

This will come in handy for some of the recipes in this cookbook!

CALORIES PER SERVING: 172

PROTEIN: 33G

CARBS: 6G

FAT: 2G

SERVES 4

1 Whole Free range roasting chicken {around 4-5lbs}

3 Carrots

2 Medium onions

3 Stalks of celery

Dried rosemary

Thyme

Salt

Pepper

Apple Cider Vinegar

Water {Around 11-12 Cups}

HOW TO MAKE:

Rinse off your chicken and put it in a big saucepan or soup pan (remove giblets and place to one side).

Chop your vegetables into large chunks.

Leave the skins on as they add to the taste and the nutrients.

Add the herbs and salt and pepper to the pan.

Add at least ¼ cup of fine sea salt to add flavor to your stock.

Fill the pan with water so that the chicken and vegetables are completely covered.

Bring to boiling point on a high heat and then reduce the heat and allow the stock to simmer for 3-4 hours.

Check at intervals and top up with water if it does not fully cover the vegetables.

Take off the heat and carefully remove the chicken, placing to one side. You now need to strain the liquid from the stockpot into another bowl using a sieve to get rid of all the lumpy bits.

Leave the stock and chicken to cool.

Once cool, tear or cut the meat from the bones. You can save the bones and make a bone broth later but get rid of the veggies.

Once cooled to room temperature, add to a sealed container and keep in the freezer. This can be kept for weeks if in an airtight Tupperware box or Kilner jar just skim off the fat when ready to use.

The rest of the chicken will taste great if added to the stock as a soup or you could enjoy it added to a crispy salad.

RED MEAT AND PORK

Meaty and manly, red meat and pork is great for bodybuilding, as well as fitting into the paleo 'okay' list. These recipes will help you look beyond the steak and egg option on your meal plan. Enjoy!

BRAWN
BISON BURGER

This brawny burger provides more than enough protein to keep you growing!

CALORIES PER SERVING: 292

PROTEIN: 43G

CARBS: 7G

FAT: 23G

MAKES 2 BURGERS

450g of ground organic bison

3 chopped jalapeno peppers

½ chopped red onion

1 finely chopped shallot

1 egg (free range)

2 crushed garlic cloves

Sprinkle of salt and pepper

HOW TO MAKE:

Pre-heat grill to a medium heat.

Cover a baking tray with foil.

Mix all of the ingredients together in a large bowl and form palm sized patties with your hands.

Place your bison patties in the middle of the baking tray and slot under the grill.

Grill patties for around 12 – 15 minutes, turning them over halfway through.

Take patties out of the grill when both sides are golden and the meat is cooked through.

Plate and serve with a side salad.

BRAWNY
BEEF LETTUCE FAJITAS

Quick and easy beef recipe, perfect for lunch and packed with loads of protein to keep you growing and burning fat

CALORIES PER SERVING: 329

PROTEIN: 35G

CARBS: 33G

FAT: 6G

HOW TO MAKE:

Add the diced steak, chopped onion, red pepper and 1 tbsp of chilli sauce to a pan on a medium heat and stir-fry for around 4 – 5 minutes.

Add the steak mix to the whole lettuce leaves.

Add one more tbsp of sweet chilli sauce and roll up like a wrap.

Plate and serve.

SERVES 1

100g of diced lean beef steak

1 chopped red onion

1 chopped red pepper

1 Cos or lambs lettuce, broken into whole leaves

2 tbsp of sweet chilli sauce

s

BULK-UP
BEEF AND BROCCOLI CURRY

This absolutely delicious curry is packed full of flavour and has a hefty dose of protein to boot.

CALORIES PER SERVING: 298

PROTEIN: 30G

CARBS: 10G

FAT: 12G

SERVES 5

450g of diced sirloin frying steak

2 tbsp of coconut oil

2 minced garlic cloves

1 tbsp of lemon juice

250ml of homemade chicken stock

2 chopped carrots

1 chopped onion

2 tbsp of grated ginger

½ broccoli

Sprinkle of salt and pepper

HOW TO MAKE:

Pre-heat the coconut oil and garlic in a large pan over a medium to high heat.

Add the diced steak and salt to the pan and brown both sides.

Once brown, take the beef out and leave to one side.

Get a bowl and mix the pepper, ginger, lemon juice and ¼ of the home-made chicken stock.

Add the broccoli, onions and chopped carrots into the pan.

Add the last of the stock over the beef and simmer for 40 minutes or until beef soft and tender..

Plate and serve.

PEPPERY
STEAK & MUSCLE MUSHROOMS

A very quick and easy paleo meal but tasty all the same.

CALORIES PER SERVING: 378

PROTEIN: 22G

CARBS: 5G

FAT: 30G

SERVES 1

250g of rib eye steak

Sprinkle of salt and pepper

2 tbsp of olive oil

1 chopped red pepper

2 minced garlic cloves

100g of white baby mushrooms

HOW TO MAKE:

Get a large frying pan and heat the olive oil on a high heat.

Pepper the steaks and add to the pan.

Fry the steaks for 6 minutes in total, turning the steaks halfway through.

Take the steak out of the pan and leave to cool.

Add the baby mushrooms, peppers and cloves to the pan and sauté for around 15 minutes or until the mushrooms become soft.

Pour the mushroom mix over the steaks.

Plate and serve.

PALEO
BEEFY STIR FRY

A very quick and easy, healthy beef stir-fry that's packed full of protein to help you build muscle and burn fat.

CALORIES PER SERVING: 277

PROTEIN: 30G

CARBS: 7G

FAT: 14G

SERVES 4

400g of diced frying beef steaks

1 broccoli, broken into florets

4 chopped celery sticks

1 corn on the cob (corn removed from the husk)

150ml organic beef or chicken stock

2 tbsp of horseradish sauce

1 tbsp of olive oil

Sprinkle of salt and pepper

HOW TO MAKE:

Heat the olive oil in a frying pan on a high heat.

Add salt and pepper to the beefsteaks and place them in the frying pan.

Stir-fry for 2 minutes until the beef is browned, then remove and set aside.

Add the broccoli and chopped celery to the pan and fry for a further 2 minutes.

Add the beef stock to the pan, then cover.

Reduce the heat and let the veg simmer for 2 minutes.

Place the steak back in the pan and mix with the other vegetables for another minute.

Plate and serve with the horseradish.

FISH AND SEAFOOD

The great thing about fish is that it is so good for you and can be used in so many different ways. It's paleo friendly, low in fat, and the omega 3 boosts your brain-power and stamina, keeping you focused on your reps and sets. Don't ignore fish as a fancy option– embrace it into your meal plan!

MUSCLE TILAPIA

Tilapia is an exotic sounding fish but can often be found in your local fishmonger or superstore counter. Failing this, you can use this recipe with tuna steaks or any other fish fillets of your choice!

CALORIES PER SERVING: 478

PROTEIN: 41G

CARBS: 9G

FAT: 32G

SERVES 1

2 Tilapia fillets (you could sway for tuna steak depending on location and sustainability lists)

3 Minced garlic cloves

1 Thumb sized piece of fresh ginger (minced)

Finely diced fresh green chilli

1 Freshly squeezed lime

2 tbsp of olive oil

HOW TO MAKE:

Heat the olive oil in a frying pan on a medium heat.

Add the ginger, chilli and garlic and soften (do not let burn or crisp by continuing to stir).

Once soft, add the fish and cook for 2-3 minutes.

Flip the fish over and cook for a further 2-3 minutes. (well-done tuna steak will need 3 more minutes on each side; keep an eye on the colour of the sides of the fish (you'll see it turn from pink to brown at the top and bottom – leave the centre pink if you like it medium).

Serve with fresh lime juice to finish and a crispy green salad.

SUPER
COD PARCELS

A simple recipe that's quick and easy to make and tasty too.

CALORIES PER SERVING: 324

PROTEIN: 28G

CARBS: 11G

FAT: 19G

SERVES 1

2x 175g cod fillets

2 sheets of grease-proof or baking paper

2 tbsp chopped flat-leaf parsley

Juice of 1 lemon

175g organic cherry tomatoes

25g olives

1 tbsp olive oil

HOW TO MAKE:

Preheat oven to (180°C /350°f/Gas Mark 4).

Tear off a square of paper and place a cod fillet in the centre.

Scatter half of the other ingredients around it and fold shut.

Repeat with the other cod fillet.

Bake for 15 minutes in the oven.

Open the parcel and squeeze more lemon juice over to serve.

Plate and serve.

TANGY SEABASS & TENDER-STEM BROCCOLI

A healthy duo to boost brainpower and strength - essential for a perfect workout..

CALORIES PER SERVING: 223

PROTEIN: 20G

CARBS: 5G

FAT: 15G

SERVES 2

2x 100g sea bass fillets (skin on)

1 bunch of tender stem broccoli (or half a head of broccoli)

2 tbsp olive oil

Juice of 1 lime

Sprinkle of salt and pepper

HOW TO MAKE:

Place a pan of water on a high heat and leave to boil.

Add the broccoli into the boiling water for 5-6 minutes.

Heat the oil in a separate pan on a medium heat and place the sea bass, skin down on to the pan. Hold the fillet for a few seconds to prevent the sides from curling up and shrinking.

Cook for 3 minutes and turn over.

Take the broccoli off the heat, drain and put to one side (check for taste first– crunchy is best but some like it softer!)

Cook the sea bass fillets for a further 2-3 minutes.

Add the lime juice to the sea bass and salt and pepper to taste.

Plate and serve the sea bass with the broccoli.

BRIT FISH AND CHIPS

A winter warmer served with chips that you're actually allowed to indulge in.

CALORIES PER SERVING: 385

PROTEIN: 25G

CARBS: 25G

FAT: 24G

SERVES 2

2 large sweet potatoes, peeled and cut into thick chips (fries)

3 tbsp olive oil

1 garlic clove, crushed

Juice of 1 lemon

2x 125g skinless white fish fillets (look for sustainably caught)

A serving of fresh green peas

Handful of finely chopped fresh mint

Sprinkle of salt and pepper

HOW TO MAKE:

Heat oven to (180°C /400°f/Gas Mark 6).

Boil a pan of water on a high heat.

Place the sweet potato fries in the pan of boiling water and leave for 10 minutes.

Drain the sweet potatoes (keep the water but turn the pan off!) and spread out on an oven dish.

Drizzle the sweet potatoes with ½ the olive oil and salt and pepper and place in the oven.

Cook the sweet potato for 15 minutes before adding the fish fillets to the dish, sprinkling with the rest of the olive oil and salt and pepper.

Allow the fish fillets to cook for 10-15 minutes or to the recommended guidelines on the packaging.

A few minutes before the fish is ready, place the peas into the pan of water and allow to boil on a high heat.

Drain the peas and add the mint.

Stir with half the squeezed lemon.

Remove the fish and chips from the oven before squeezing the rest of the lemon over the fish.

A last sprinkle of salt and pepper to taste.

Plate and serve and enjoy your British classic the paleo way!

LANGOUSTINE AND RED PEPPER RICE-FREE PAELLA

A Mediterranean Masterpiece.

SERVES 2

3 tbsp olive oil

2 red peppers, cut into cubes (about ½ cm thick)

Handful of black olives

1 zucchini (courgette) cut into cubes about ½ cm thick

1 tbsp paprika

7 large organic tomatoes cut into eight pieces

300g langoustines - butterflied

1 fresh lemon, cut into quarters

1 serving of cooked fresh peas

HOW TO MAKE:

Heat oven to (150°C /300°f/Gas Mark 2).

Oil a baking tray and add the tomatoes, pepper, olives and zucchini.

Drizzle a little more olive oil over the vegetables and sprinkle salt and pepper and paprika over the top.

Oven bake for 30-40 minutes.

Whilst your vegetable mix is roasting, butterfly your langoustines:

Pull off the head and legs with your fingers and leave the tails for presentation.

Score down the centre of each prawn (do not slice in half) and then pull open on each side of the score to flatten.

Turn the oven up to (180°C /350°f/Gas Mark 4) and add your prawns to a roasting tray, drizzle with olive oil.

Cook for 6-7 minutes, ensuring piping hot before serving.

Serve the roasted vegetables (with added peas) in a pasta/rice dish with the prawns on top and the lemon wedges for squeezing.

Add salt and pepper to taste.

SUPER
HUMAN MACKEREL & BRAWNY BEETROOT

A delicious mackerel meal - packed full of protein and super-charged beetroot.

CALORIES PER SERVING: 375

PROTEIN: 25G

CARBS: 20G

FAT: 30G

SERVES 2

175g skinned sweet potatoes

200g smoked mackerel fillets, skin removed

4 spring onions, finely sliced

140g small cooked beetroot, sliced into wedges

Small bunch dill, finely chopped

1 tsp caraway seeds

2 tbsp olive oil
Juice 1 lemon, zest of half

HOW TO MAKE:

Bring a pan of water to the boil on a high heat.

Add the potatoes and simmer for 15 minutes or until fork-tender.

Drain and cool and cut into thick slices.

Flake the mackerel into a bowl and add the cooled potatoes, spring onions, beetroot and dill.

In a separate bowl, whisk together the olive oil, lemon juice, caraway seeds and some seasoning.

Pour the dressing over the mackerel salad and toss everything to coat.

Scatter over the lemon zest.

Pack into plastic containers and chill, or eat straight away.

Plate and serve.

CATCH
OF THE DAY

A wild and fresh treat.

CALORIES PER SERVING: 504

PROTEIN: 36G

CARBS: 17G

FAT: 33G

SERVES 1

1 whole trout cleaned and gutted (best caught yourself! If fishing doesn't come naturally, make sure it's sustainable)

2 green peppers, deseeded and chopped

8 cherry tomatoes halved

Handful of cilantro (coriander)

Handful of parsley

1 fresh lemon

1 clove minced garlic

1 tbsp olive oil,

Sprinkle of salt and pepper

HOW TO MAKE:

Heat oven to (190°C /375°f/Gas Mark 5).

Stuff the trout with the fresh herbs (save a handful for garnish), olive oil, and garlic.

Add to an oiled baking tray, surrounded by the vegetables.

Cook for 10-15 minutes – the fish must be piping hot before serving.

Serve with the lemon chunks and garnish with a handful of leftover herbs.
.

SUPER STRONG SALMON FRITTATAS

A tasty paleo meal that will keep you building muscle and burning fat!

CALORIES PER SERVING: 340

PROTEIN: 25G

CARBS: 15G

FAT: 20G

SERVES 4

2x 125g wild salmon fillets

1 head of broccoli (pull off the florets)

1 tbsp olive oil

Handful of cilantro (coriander) and parsley

8 free range eggs, beaten

2 large peeled, sweet potatoes.

HOW TO MAKE:

Bring a pan of water to the boil on a high heat and add the sweet potatoes, cook for 20 minutes.

Steam the salmon over the pan for the last 15 minutes.

Add the broccoli in the same pan as the potatoes for the last 4-5 minutes of cooking and then drain.

Use your fork to flake the cooked salmon into a separate bowl whilst the potatoes and broccoli are cooling.

Use a knife to roughly chop the sweet potato into thin slices.

Mix the broccoli, sweet potato and salmon.

Heat the olive oil in a pan on a medium heat.

Add the potato and broccoli and salmon in a large omelette shape.

Mix eggs with herbs and pour over the ingredients.

Cook on a medium heat for 6-7 minutes (once edges are brown and a little crispy use a flat spatula to lift from the base of the pan and prevent sticking).

Continue to cook on a low heat for a further 5 minutes or until frittata can be easily lifted from the pan with your spatula.

Serve on a bed of salad!

TRAINING THAI BROTH

An Asian take on bodybuilding feasts.

CALORIES PER SERVING: 440

PROTEIN: 40G

CARBS: 25G

FAT: 20G

SERVES 4

2x 125g skinless cod pieces

2 tbsp olive oil

1 tbsp coriander seeds

2 fresh limes

1 garlic clove

1 thumb size piece of minced ginger

1 white onion, chopped

50g spinach leaves

Handful of fresh basil leaves

1 pak choi

125ml of homemade chicken stock

125ml of good quality organic coconut milk (if available)

1 small green pepper deseeded and finely chopped

2 stems of spring onion, chopped

HOW TO MAKE:

Crush the fresh herbs and spices in a blender or use a pestle and mortar.

Mix in to 1 tbsp of olive oil until a paste is formed.

Heat a large pan or wok with sesame oil on a high heat.

Fry the onions, garlic and ginger until soft but not crispy or browned.

Add the spice paste with the coconut milk and stir.

Slowly add the stock until a broth is formed.

Now add your fish pieces and allow to simmer in the broth for 10-15 minutes.

Add the pak choi leaves 2-3 minutes before the end of the cooking time.

Plate and serve hot with the chilli and spring onion sprinkled over the top.

STEAMY PALEO WORKOUT FISH

This dish is fresh and delicious; it's so easy to cook and you can cram it full with extra greens and vitamins!

CALORIES PER SERVING: 208

PROTEIN: 20G

CARBS: 5G

FAT: 12G

SERVES 4

2x 140g trout fillets

4 rectangles of tin foil or baking paper

1 large red pepper, deseeded and chopped

2 large tomatoes, roughly chopped

1 garlic clove, chopped

1 tbsp olive oil, plus a little extra

1 tbsp balsamic vinegar

2 tbsp flaked almonds

25g arugula (rocket)

1 lime cut into wedges

HOW TO MAKE:

Heat oven to (200°C /400°f/Gas Mark 6).

Cut off four large rectangles and place each fillet on each piece of paper.

Mix the balsamic vinegar, ½ lime juice, red pepper, tomatoes, garlic, almonds and olive oil in a separate bowl.

Drizzle generously over each trout fillet.

Fold these up into a parcel leaving one edge open.

Cook for 20 minutes then add the spring onions and chilli for a fresh taste to end.

Plate and serve with the remaining lime wedges.

VEGETARIAN RECIPES

While everyone knows that in order to build muscle, a diet rich in protein is necessary to supplement exercises and/or gym workouts, many people think that animal meat is the only rich source of protein. This is a myth. There are lots of veggies out there that are good, and even better, substitutes for meat.

The fact is, a vegetarian diet can also work for muscle building and in a much healthier way. For one, the risk of contracting heart disease, hypertension, diabetes, and other serious health conditions that are usually associated with consumption of meat products are definitely lessened.

This section will show you how you can whip up recipes that are not only healthy but are also easy to prepare; saving you a lot of precious time. In today's busy world, the ability to prepare quick and healthy meals will give you a decided advantage when working on your goals.

So, who says that a tasty vegetarian meal and muscle building do not go together? With this book, you will discover that it is possible. Read on and find out how.

BREAKFAST

Everyone knows that breakfast is the most important meal of the day. Since childhood, you've been told that you need to have a hearty breakfast to start your day and to provide you with enough energy to face the tasks ahead. That is absolutely true – especially if you are aiming to build muscle. Without proper nutrition, how can you expect your body to endure the tough grind at the gym?

As a bodybuilder, you need a sufficient amount of protein as well as the right amount of essential minerals and nutrients. Thus, for a vegetarian, breakfast is also the most difficult meal to prepare. Other than eggs (for ovo or ovo-lacto vegetarians), where will you get your protein requirements? These 25 appetizing and easy to prepare breakfast recipes have the answer!

MUSCLE
FRUIT & NUT PROTEIN CEREAL

Some vegetarians are deficient in omega 3 fatty acids that are sourced primarily from fish. This recipe will address that problem and provide all the benefits from healthy fat.

CALORIES PER SERVING: 450

PROTEIN: 18G

CARBS: 55G

FAT: 21G

HOW TO MAKE:

Get a small bowl and combine all the dry ingredients.

Pour the cashew milk on top. Serve immediately.

SERVES 1

- 2 tbsp of dried apricots
- 1 scoop of vanilla protein powder
- 1 tbsp of flaked almonds
- 1 tbsp of dried raisins
- 1 tbsp of Chia seeds
- 1 tbsp of buckwheat
- 1 tbsp of hemp seeds
- 1 tbsp of dried cranberries
- 175ml of cashew milk

LEAN & MEAN
VEGGIE BURGER

This is the perfect on-the-go meal for the busy bodybuilder.

CALORIES PER SERVING: 441

PROTEIN: 27G

CARBS: 16G

FAT: 14G

HOW TO MAKE:

Fry the veggie burger patty in a pan on a medium heat for 7-10 minutes.

Fry the egg in the same pan for 3-4 minutes.

Prepare the roll with the egg and spinach topping the burger.

Serve and enjoy.

SERVES 1

2 regular-sized eggs

Handful of baby spinach leaves

1 whole wheat roll

1 veggie burger patty

COCONUT
POWERED PANCAKES

Providing a new twist to the traditional home-cooked breakfast favourite, this recipe is light on the tummy but packs enough protein for muscle building.

CALORIES PER SERVING: 323

PROTEIN: 22G

CARBS: 25G

FAT: 15G

HOW TO MAKE:

Pre-heat a skillet over medium to high heat.

Blend all the ingredients together. Pour roughly ½ cup of the pancake batter into the pan and cook for 1-2 minutes. Flip the pancake and cook for another 30 seconds. Once done, remove your tasty pancake. Use the same method for the rest of your batter.

Serve and enjoy immediately.

SERVES 2

4 egg whites

2 tbsp of coconut flour

1 tsp of cinnamon

1 scoop of vanilla protein powder

1 diced regular-sized banana

Handful of walnuts

Handful of almonds

1 dash of cinnamon

2 tbsp honey

RIPPED & READY PANCAKES

Even without slathering your plate with sweet syrup, these pancakes are already tasty and sweet as they are

```
CALORIES PER SERVING: 315

PROTEIN: 19G

CARBS: 35G

FAT: 11
```

SERVES 1

50g gluten free flour

4 egg whites

1/2 tsp of baking powder

1 tbsp of blueberries

1 tbsp of walnuts

HOW TO MAKE:

Pre-heat the skillet over medium to high heat.

Blend all the ingredients together. Pour roughly ½ cup of the pancake batter into the pan and cook for 1-2 minutes. Flip the pancake and cook for another 30 seconds. Once done, remove your tasty pancake. Use the same method for the rest of your batter.

Serve and enjoy immediately.

BRAWNY APPLE, KALE & BLUEBERRY SMOOTHIE

If you love having a fruit smoothie for breakfast, why not add some kale to your drink and spike up your breakfast with plenty of health benefits? Quick and easy to prepare, you won't even taste the veggies in your drink.

CALORIES PER SERVING: 312

PROTEIN: 27

CARBS: 42

FAT: 4

HOW TO MAKE:

Combine all the ingredients together in a blender and process until smooth consistency is achieved.

Serve immediately and enjoy.

SERVES 1

100g of kale

1 chopped and halved apple

100g of frozen blueberries

1 scoop of vanilla protein powder

1/2 tbsp of unsweetened almond milk

1 to 2 ice cubes

OAT
MUSCLE MUSH

Mush for breakfast? Why Not? As long as you get the nutrients you need to jumpstart your day, there should be no problem – and this gives a boost and more!

CALORIES PER SERVING: 536

PROTEIN: 33G

CARBS: 74G

FAT: 14G

HOW TO MAKE:

Get a small bowl and combine all the ingredients.

Heat in the microwave oven for 1 or 2 minutes, or until the oats have absorbed all the liquid.

Add the strawberries and almond butter to the top.

Serve and enjoy.

SERVES 1

100g of oatmeal

4 egg whites

1 tsp of honey

2 tbsp of unsweetened almond milk

1/2 scoop of Chocolate protein powder

4 diced strawberries

1 tbsp of almond butter

BRAWNY
VEGGIE SAUSAGE CLUB

Who says vegetarians miss out on homemade breakfast classics like this? With a little creativity, vegetarians don't have to miss anything – except the meat!

CALORIES PER SERVING: 472

PROTEIN: 42G

CARBS: 32G

FAT: 21G

SERVES 1

2 large veggie sausage patties

2 large eggs

1 slice of whole grain bread

50g spinach leaves

HOW TO MAKE:

Bring a pan of water to the boil and add a dash of white wine vinegar and salt. Reduce the heat and crack the eggs in, allowing to float as it is in the water. Cook for 3 minutes (check that the whites are opaque).

While the eggs are cooking, heat a frying pan with some vegetable oil and lightly fry the veggie patties until heated through.

Toss in the spinach to wilt at the last minute.

Serve with the toasted wholegrain bread.

POACHED EGGS
WITH SUPER SPINACH & KALE

You could expect to be served this dish in any top restaurant; poached eggs make anything posh and they're also probably the healthiest way of cooking your eggs to make the most of all that protein.

CALORIES PER SERVING: 170

PROTEIN: 15G

CARBS: 5G

FAT: 10G

SERVES 2

4 medium-sized eggs

50g kale (stems removed)

50g baby spinach

1 tbsp of olive oil

1 tbsp of white wine vinegar

1 crushed and finely chopped garlic clove

Sprinkle of salt

Sprinkle of pepper

HOW TO MAKE:

Heat olive oil in a skillet on a medium heat and add the garlic.

Toss in kale and sauté until wilted or for about 2 to 3 minutes. Transfer the kale onto a plate and set aside.

Boil water in a large pot. Once it boils, reduce the heat and add 1 tbsp of white wine vinegar.

Crack the eggs in and allow to cook until for about 3 minutes or when the egg whites are not translucent anymore.

Remove the eggs and lay on top of the kale and baby spinach.

Sprinkle with a dash of salt & pepper to taste.

Serve and enjoy while hot.

ALMOND-CHOCO QUINOA

A filling and tasty breakfast or evening snack, the all-time favourite chocolate and peanut butter combo is just the thing to prime you up for a workout-heavy day.

CALORIES PER SERVING: 375

PROTEIN: 15

CARBS: 45

FAT: 15

HOW TO MAKE:

Put the almond milk and quinoa together in a pan and heat on a low setting.

Cover the pan to allow the quinoa to cook well for around 15 minutes, stirring frequently.

While still warm, stir in the protein powder, peanut butter, and add maple syrup or honey to serve for a little extra something!

SERVES 2

360ml unsweetened almond milk

125g of quinoa

3 tbsp of crunchy almond butter

1 heaped tbsp of chocolate protein powder

1 tbsp of honey

BULKY
BREAKFAST TORTILLA

A "meaty" and satisfying breakfast, it is nutrient-rich too – but without the meat!

CALORIES PER SERVING: 537

PROTEIN: 37

CARBS: 34

FAT: 27

SERVES 1

2 eggs

1 wholegrain tortilla

2 tbsp of soy milk

1/4 of onion, chopped

2 oz of vegetarian sausage

35g of low-fat cheddar cheese, grated

3 tbsp of olive oil

HOW TO MAKE:

Heat 1 tbsp of cooking oil in a skillet.

Sauté onions for 2 minutes.

In a small bowl, mix the beaten egg with the milk and season to taste.

Pour the mix into the skillet, stirring with a cooking spoon to scramble the egg and then set aside on a warm plate.

Heat 1 tbsp of cooking oil in the same skillet.

Cook the sausage until brown, crumbling the "meat" while stirring.

Combine the egg and sausage on the tortilla.

Top with cheese and roll to make a burrito – fold at the bottom so you don't drip it all over your gym clothes.

BRAWNY
BREAKFAST WITH TEMPEH & POTATO

If you enjoy vegetarian hash browns, you will definitely like this tempeh version. It is filling, and tastes amazing.

CALORIES PER SERVING: 324

PROTEIN: 24G

CARBS: 37G

FAT: 12G

SERVES 1

½ packet of tempeh, diced into 1/2" cubes

2 medium sized potatoes, diced

1 tbsp of soy sauce

1 ½ tbsp olive oil

½ onion, diced

50g of baby spinach

½ garlic clove, finely choped

1 pinch of salt & pepper

HOW TO MAKE:

Put the potatoes in a pot of water, making sure they are fully submerged. Cover the pot, and bring to a boil. Allow the potatoes to sit in boiling water for at least 10 minutes or until they become tender. Remove from pot and drain well.

Heat a skillet and sauté onions, tempeh, and potatoes in soy sauce and olive oil. Stir frequently to make sure that the tempeh cubes are cooked well on all sides. Drizzle with garlic and salt & pepper and place on a bed of baby spinach.

Serve and enjoy.

VEGGIE BREAKFAST BURRITO

A fast alternative to your average morning start; these burritos are loaded with healthy goodness, just waiting to turn into the energy you need for the rest of the day.

CALORIES PER SERVING: 350

PROTEIN: 25G

CARBS: 40G

FAT: 10G

SERVES 3

3 medium eggs, whisked lightly

1 tsp olive oil

2 wholegrain flour tortillas (

½ white onion, finely chopped

½ can mixed beans

A pinch of salt & pepper

1 tsp of ketchup

1 tbsp natural yoghurt

1 tsp cayenne pepper

HOW TO MAKE:

Heat the olive oil in a non-stick skillet.

Season the eggs with salt & pepper then pour over the skillet once the oil is hot.

Now add the onions and stir occasionally with the eggs until the eggs are cooked. Turn off the heat just before they're fully cooked through if you like your eggs creamy, otherwise continue until fully cooked and white.

Meanwhile add the mixed beans to a separate pan with a little tomato ketchup, heating through for 3-5 minutes.

Divide the cooked egg in half and spoon each part with half of the beans into each tortilla.

Dollop half of the natural yoghurt and a sprinkle of cayenne pepper on each mix.

Wrap the tortillas. Serve warm.

MIGHTY MUFFINS
WITH VANILLA AND BLUEBERRIES

This light breakfast is ideal on your rest days in-between workouts. Light on carbs, it is packed with protein to help in muscle building even when resting.

CALORIES PER SERVING: 190

PROTEIN: 15

CARBS: 3

FAT: 3

SERVES 1

1 scoop of Whey Protein (vanilla flavour)

3 egg whites

35g of oat flour

1 tbsp coconut flour

1 tsp of baking powder

1 tsp of salt

1 tsp stevia

25g fresh blueberries

HOW TO MAKE:

Pre-heat the oven to (325°F/170 °C/Gas Mark 3).

Mix all of the ingredients in a mixing bowl.

Divide the batter into quarters and spoon into a cake/cookie tin.

Place in the oven and bake for 15-20 minutes, using a knife to test whether they're cooked or not (gently slot into the middle of one of the buns – the knife should pull out clean).

Remove and cool on a rack before serving alone or with a blob of natural yoghurt and some extra fresh fruit!

BRAWNY
CHOCO BANANA AND ALMOND OATMEAL

This is a great recipe for people who are in a rush to get to work. In 5 minutes, you can whip up this sustaining and healthy meal that contains all the essential nutrients your body needs.

CALORIES PER SERVING: 523

PROTEIN: 32G

CARBS: 60G

FAT: 15G

SERVES 1

50 grams of rolled oats

200ml of almond milk

1 scoop of chocolate whey protein (or vanilla, if preferred)

A handful of almonds (chopped or flaked)

1 diced medium-sized banana

1tsp of organic peanut butter

HOW TO MAKE:

Mash the banana with a fork in a separate bowl.

Mix the protein powder with the oats.

Pour the almond milk into a pan on a low to medium heat and once bubbling add the rolled oats and protein.

Turn the heat down and simmer, throwing in the almonds, banana and peanut butter.

Stir often to prevent the oats from sticking.

Once heated through, turn off the heat and serve,

SPICY MUSCLE
TOFU & CHILLI SPINACH SCRAMBLE

An easy to prepare recipe that packs a lot of protein and amino acids the body needs, not to mention a lot of spice. This is also very easy to prepare..

CALORIES PER SERVING: 270

PROTEIN: 25G

CARBS: 20G

FAT: 10G

SERVES 2

225g of extra-firm tofu, chopped into chunks

50g spinach leaves

50g of sliced mushrooms

50g cup of cherry tomatoes

1tsp of lemon juice

1 tsp of olive oil

1 clove of fresh garlic, finely chopped

1 tsp of light soy sauce,

1 tsp of red chilli flakes or finely chopped fresh chilli

A pinch of salt & pepper

HOW TO MAKE:

Heat the olive oil in a skillet over a medium heat.

Add the mushrooms, tomatoes and garlic. Fry until mushrooms are soft and golden brown.

Lower the heat and add the tofu, lemon juice, soy sauce, and salt & pepper. Cook for 3 to 5 minutes.

Turn the heat off and add the spinach, allowing it to wilt.

Serve with chilli and salt and pepper.

Serve with pre-cooked quinoa (see chapter 4 – Sides for Sweet Cinnamon Quinoa recipe, if preferred).

).

AESTHETIC TOFU & SPRING ONION SCRAMBLE

A crisp and fresh version of your scrambled eggs on toast!

CALORIES PER SERVING: 343

PROTEIN: 25G

CARBS: 30G

FAT: 22G

SERVES 2

225g of extra firm tofu, pressed and crumbled

1 tbsp of olive oil

3 stems of spring onion finely chopped

50g spinach leaves

5 cherry tomatoes, quartered

1 clove of garlic, finely chopped

1/2 tsp of Worcestershire sauce

1 tsp of lemon juice

2 slices of whole grain bread

HOW TO MAKE:

Heat olive oil in a frying pan over a medium heat setting.

Toss in the spring onion, tomatoes and garlic.

Lower the heat and add the tofu, lemon juice, Worcestershire sauce, and salt & pepper.

Cook for 3 to 5 minutes.

Turn the heat off and add the spinach.

Transfer to a serving dish.

Serve with toasted bread and enjoy

PROTEIN-PACKED TOFU SCRAMBLE

Feel free to experiment with your left over veggies for this one. The nutritional yeast actually makes this dish taste a little like cheese, so you can enjoy the home comfort without the dairy guilt.

CALORIES PER SERVING: 250

PROTEIN: 24

CARBS: 9G

FAT: 8G

SERVES 4

1 tbsp olive oil

225g of firm tofu

2 tbsp of nutritional yeast

1 slice of veggie bacon substitute (made from tempeh), chopped

¼ tsp of turmeric

1 tsp of light soy sauce

1 stalk of broccoli, chopped into small pieces

¼ red pepper, chopped

½ onion, finely chopped

1 dash of cayenne pepper

Pinch of black pepper

30g spinach leaves

HOW TO MAKE:

Drain and press the tofu well before cutting into chunks.

Get a mixing bowl and put the tofu pieces in. Add the turmeric, soy sauce, nutritional yeast, pepper, and cayenne. Use a fork to mash it all together, ending with an almost smooth texture.

Cover everything in plastic wrap. Put in the refrigerator and leave overnight if you have time (if not don't worry, you'll still have a tasty dish).

When ready to cook, heat the olive oil in a skillet on a medium heat and fry the "bacon" until crispy and brown.

Stir in the veggies, frying until soft.

Add the tofu and fry for a further 3-5 minutes, mixing well.

Serve with a side of raw spinach leaves for extra protein.

Serve and enjoy!

PEANUT BUTTER AND BANANA CEREAL WRAP

A childhood favourite – peanut butter and banana – still tastes just as great as you remember and considering this is packed with protein and fibre, I say it's an indulgence you can afford.

CALORIES PER SERVING: 639

PROTEIN: 18G

CARBS: 82G

FAT: 28G

HOW TO MAKE:

Spread 2 tbsp of peanut butter on the tortilla. Lay the bananas and granola on top of the peanut butter.

Wrap the tortilla.

Add honey or maple syrup as an occasional treat.

Breakfast is done.

SERVES 1

2 tbsp of peanut butter

1 banana, thinly sliced

1 wholegrain tortilla

50g granola

BRAWNY BREAKFAST

When you feel the need for your comforting toast, this is the delicious healthy option to go for..

CALORIES PER SERVING: 509

PROTEIN: 23

CARBS: 36

FAT: 30

SERVES 1

1 tsp olive oil

2 slices of Ezekiel bread (or gluten free)

½ very ripe avocado

2 eggs

½ red pepper, diced

Pinch of salt and pepper

Pinch of sunflower or chia seeds

HOW TO MAKE:

Remove the skin from the avocado (wrapping half tightly in cling film for later). Mix the avocado with the red pepper and salt and pepper.

Add the Ezekiel bread to the toaster.

Lightly fry the eggs in a little olive oil (have poached for an even healthier option).

Spread the avocado mix on to the toast, topping with the fried eggs and sprinkle with the seeds to serve.

ENTRÉES

Once breakfast is done, all we're thinking about is our workout and then our next meal. The dishes I include in this section are a variety of my favourite meals as they are delicious and packed with as much protein as possible. You really don't need to miss out as a vegetarian and anyone who says that vegetarian bodybuilding is not possible… well they need to think again. Using a combination of seeds, vegetables and plant based products as well as healthy dairy options, protein need not be the taboo word of the Veggie world. While protein is important, we also need a diet rich in vitamins and minerals and so these dishes seek to provide a balanced combination of all these goodies – I've done the hard work here so you don't need to. Just buy the ingredients and get cooking! You can't argue with spending less time on your meal plans and more time lifting weights now can you?

MUSCLE
MUSHROOM WITH TOFU & QUINOA

A meaty mushroom flavor packed full of protein to keep your energy levels high and your motivation moving!

CALORIES PER SERVING: 366

PROTEIN: 20G

CARBS: 40G

FAT: 14G

SERVES 2

2 large Portabella mushrooms (dried and rinsed clean)	2 cherry tomatoes, sliced	1 crushed garlic clove, finely chopped
	½ onion, diced	
75g of cooked quinoa	1 tbsp of shredded non-fat mozzarella cheese	¼ tbsp of onion powder
50g of baby spinach		¼ tbsp of cumin
50g of kale	½ tbsp olive oil	Pinch of salt & pepper to taste
225g of firm or extra firm tofu, press and crumble well	¼ tbsp of paprika	

HOW TO MAKE:

Turn the grill on to high.

Get a large sauté pan and heat olive oil on a medium heat.

Toss in the tofu, kale and diced onion and sauté for around 3 minutes or until the onion starts to soften.

Add the spices, salt & pepper, and quinoa. Sauté for a couple of minutes more.

Place the portabello mushrooms on a baking sheet and lightly brush with olive oil. Stack the mushroom cap with quinoa mixture, spinach, shredded cheese, and sliced tomatoes.

Grill for another 5 minutes, and then serve immediately. Enjoy!

TASTY
TEMPEH RICE BOWL

This protein-packed recipe is great for lunch or dinner on a regular day. Use the leftover veggies in the fridge and give them an exciting twist with some creativity.

CALORIES PER SERVING: 246

PROTEIN: 23G

CARBS: 94G

FAT: 13G

SERVES 1

75g of tempeh (crumbled)

150g of cooked brown rice

8 cherry tomatoes, diced

½ red bell pepper, sliced

½ green bell pepper, sliced

1 tbsp of soy sauce

½ tsp of ginger

½ tsp of onion powder

1 garlic clove, finely diced & crushed

½ tsp of chilli paste

1 sliced green onion

HOW TO MAKE:

Put some olive oil in a large-sized sauté pan and heat over medium setting.

Toss in the bell peppers, tomatoes and onion and stir until softened lightly.

Add the rest of the ingredients to the pan apart from the tempeh and the rice.

Get another pan and pre-heat over medium setting. Add the tempeh.

Allow to cook for around 5 minutes. Stir from time to time.

Put brown rice in a bowl and top with tempeh, green onions, and other veggies. Serve hot and enjoy!

SPEEDY
BLACK BEAN SURPRISE

If you're craving the distinct taste of an authentic Mexican meal, this recipe can solve your problem –
without the usual grease that comes hand in hand with the takeaway version!

CALORIES PER SERVING: 550

PROTEIN: 25G

CARBS: 90G

FAT: 10G

HOW TO MAKE:

Get a big bowl and mix all the ingredients together.

Enjoy your authentic Mexican meal.

SERVES 1

50g of freshly cooked brown rice

50g of freshly cooked quinoa

50g of freshly cooked bulghar wheat

Handful of black olives

75g of cooked black beans

¼ avocado, sliced

2 tbsp of plain non-fat Greek yogurt

2 tbsp of salsa

A generous dash of hot sauce

BRAWNY VEG LASAGNA

Very low in fat and vegan, this is a quick and easy to prepare crockpot meal using only a few ingredients and very filling too!

CALORIES PER SERVING: 355

PROTEIN: 20G

CARBS: 50G

FAT: 15G

SERVES 2

½ pack of soft tofu

½ pack of firm tofu

140g of whole wheat lasagne sheets (1/2 box)

100g of baby spinach

4 tbsp of almond milk

¼ tsp of garlic powder

Juice of ½ a lemon

1 ½ tbsp of fresh basil, chopped

1 can of chopped tomatoes

Black pepper to taste

1 diced courgette/zucchini

½ tsp of salt

HOW TO MAKE:

Preheat oven to (325°F/170 °C/Gas Mark 3).

Process the soft and firm tofu, garlic powder, almond milk, basil, lemon juice and salt in a blender until smooth. Toss in the spinach and courgette.

Put about 1/3 of chopped tomatoes at the bottom of an oven dish.

Top the sauce with 1/3 of the lasagne sheets and 1/3 of the spinach/tofu mixture. Repeat the layers finishing with the chopped tomatoes on top.

Cook for around 1 hour or until the pasta sheets are soft.

BRAWNY
BLACK BEAN & COTTAGE CHEESE FAJITA

A taste of the classic Mexican dish, but with a vegetarian twist, this dish is just as appetizing but a lot healthier.

CALORIES PER SERVING: 412

PROTEIN: 25G

CARBS: 60G

FAT: 8G

SERVES 2

150g of cooked and washed black beans

75g of cannellini beans, cooked

75g of red kidney beans, cooked

1 green pepper, sliced

1 yellow pepper, sliced

1 onion, sliced

1 beef tomato, chopped

75g of cottage cheese

1 packet of fajita seasoning

4 whole wheat flour tortillas

2 tbsp salsa

2 tbsp of olive oil

HOW TO MAKE:

Preheat the oven to (250°F/130 °C/Gas Mark 1/2).

In a pan on a medium heat, sauté the onions and peppers for around 2 to 4 minutes. Stir often and make sure not to overcook.

Add to the black beans and transfer to a oven proof dish.

Keep the dish warm by placing it in the oven as you prepare the other ingredients.

Dice the tomato and set aside.

Microwave the tortillas to slightly heat them up.

Assemble the fajitas.

Serve and enjoy!

VEGGIE
BRAWN BURGER

Think you can eat a wholesome burger any more? Well, try this burger recipe and it is guaranteed to convince you.

CALORIES PER SERVING: 162

PROTEIN: 26G

CARBS: 40G

FAT: 13G

SERVES 1

110g of extra firm tempah

1 tsp of red chilli flakes

½ tbsp of Sriracha (hot chilli sauce)

1 diced red pepper

¼ piece of small sized red onion

Handful of baby spinach

½ tbsp of teriyaki marinade

1 whole wheat bun

HOW TO MAKE:

Heat the grill, and then marinate the tempah in Sriracha, red chilli flakes and teriyaki marinade.

Sauté the onion in a pan on a medium heat until it is caramelized. Stir in the pepper and baby spinach for a further 3-4 minutes.

Grill the tempah for around 4 minutes on each side.

Lay down the tempah in the bun and then add the caramelized onion, spinach and diced peppers.

Serve immediately while hot. Enjoy!

TOFU
LETTUCE WRAPS

Tasty and easy to prepare, this is will make a great on-the-go lunch.

CALORIES PER SERVING: 190

PROTEIN: 18

CARBS: 12

FAT: 10

SERVES 2

½ pack of tofu, crumbled

1 head leaf lettuce

½ piece of small onion, chopped

½ piece of red bell pepper, chopped

½ tbsp of garlic, chopped

½ tbsp of olive oil

½ tbsp of soy sauce

½ tsp of ginger powder

½ tsp of onion powder

½ tsp of garlic powder

HOW TO MAKE:

Get a large pan and heat olive oil over a medium heat setting.

Sauté tofu, onion, and bell pepper for about 3-4 minutes.

Put the soy sauce and other spices into the pan and allow sauté for 2 minutes more.

Add the tofu mix to the lettuce leaves.

Serve while hot.

BLACK BEAN VEGGIE BURGERS

Tasty and easy to make – two qualities that every busy vegetarian bodybuilder loves. These veggie burgers are wholesome and satisfying.

CALORIES PER SERVING: 337

PROTEIN: 18G

CARBS: 55G

FAT: 11G

SERVES 2

½ onion, chopped

150g of black beans, well drained

75g of flour

1 slice of bread, crumbled into bread crumbs

½ tsp of seasoned salt

1 tsp of onion powder

1 tsp of garlic powder

Pinch of salt & pepper to taste

1 tsp of olive oil

HOW TO MAKE:

In a pan over a medium heat, sautee the onions for 3 to 5 minutes or until soft.

Mash the beans in a large bowl until almost smooth, then add the sautéed onion, salt, breadcrumbs, onion powder, and garlic powder. Mix well to combine.

Add flour, 1 or 2 tbsp at a time. The mixture will thicken.

Shape into patties, about ½" thick.

Fry patties in a little oil at medium-low heat setting until lightly browned and firm on each side.

Make the burgers and serve.

SPICY
SEITAN STRIPS

Seitan is a chewy, protein-rich vegetarian option and adds a chunky texture and moreish flavour to this dish.

CALORIES PER SERVING: 138

PROTEIN: 20G

CARBS: 10G

FAT: 2G

SERVES 4

340g of seitan, sliced

1 tsp of onion powder

1 tbsp of cayenne pepper

2 tsp of garlic powder

dash of hot sauce

50g of baby spinach

2 tbsp of olive oil

HOW TO MAKE:

Coat the seitan with onion powder and garlic powder.

Fry in olive oil for 5 to 7 minutes at medium-high heat setting.

Get a medium bowl, and mix the hot sauce with the seitan in the bowl.

Coat well by stirring.

Serve on a bed of baby spinach.

FETA & BRAWNY BARLEY STUFFED PORTABELLAS

This is a unique and healthy entree recipe for vegetarians in need of a high-fiber, high-protein meal..

CALORIES PER SERVING: 322

PROTEIN: 25

CARBS: 33

FAT: 10

SERVES 2

4 large portabella mushrooms

75g of cooked quinoa

100g of feta cheese, crumbled

1 red bell pepper, chopped

1 chopped beef tomato

375ml of water

½ cucumber, chopped

1 green onion, sliced

4 tsp of olive oil

1 tbsp of Dijon mustard

1 tbsp of white wine vinegar

Pinch of salt and pepper

HOW TO MAKE:

Preheat the grill.

Combine the cooked quinoa, bell pepper, feta, cucumber, green onion, mustard, white wine vinegar in a medium-sized bowl.

Place the portabella mushrooms on a baking sheet and lightly brush with olive oil. Stack the mushroom caps with the quinoa mixture.

Place under the grill for 5 minutes, then serve immediately.

Enjoy!

RUSTIC
GARLIC PROTEIN QUINOA

While this is a basic and simple recipe, it is flexible and can be modified to include other veggies or leftovers; you can also add tofu for more protein.

CALORIES PER SERVING: 292

PROTEIN: 15G

CARBS: 40G

FAT: 8

HOW TO MAKE:

Sautee garlic and onion in olive oil in a pan at medium heat until onions soften. Lower heat.

Add the quinoa and vegetable broth. Cover the pan and simmer for around 15 to 20 minutes or until quinoa is soft and liquid is significantly absorbed.

Top with cheese and beans and serve with salt to taste.

SERVES 3

25g of mozzarella cheese

50g of cooked kidney beans

100g of uncooked quinoa

500ml of vegetable broth

1 onion, diced

4 cloves of garlic, minced

1/4 tsp of salt

1 tbsp olive oil

JASON'S
SUN DRIED TOMATO & WALNUT PENNE PASTA

If you love sun-dried tomatoes, then you will definitely enjoy this gourmet pasta dish.

CALORIES PER SERVING: 375

PROTEIN: 20

CARBS: 40

FAT: 15

SERVES 4

225g of whole-wheat pasta

2 cloves of garlic, minced

50g of walnuts, coarsely chopped

75g of sun-dried tomatoes, drained & chopped, in oil

2 tbsp of olive oil

1 tsp of basil

100g of low-fat mozzarella cheese

Pinch of salt

HOW TO MAKE:

Boil a large saucepan of water.

Add the pasta and cook following directions on the package.

While the pasta is cooking, prepare the sauce. Put minced garlic in a bowl.

Add sun-dried tomatoes, walnuts, basil, mozzarella and oil.

Once the pasta is cooked, drain it and add to the sauce.

Toss through until the pasta is well coated.

Transfer the dish onto a serving plate.

Serve.

VEGETARIAN DELI SANDWICH

This is a healthy on-the-go lunch for vegetarian bodybuilders. Packed with protein and fibre, this recipe is simple and easy to prepare.

CALORIES PER SERVING: 570

PROTEIN: 26G

CARBS: 70G

FAT: 22G

HOW TO MAKE:

Get one slice of bread and put hummus on 1 side.

Put the lettuce and avocado and tomato on the top.

Top with the other bread slice.

Serve and enjoy.

SERVES 1

4 tbsp of hummus

2 tbsp of chia seeds

Handful of baby spinach

1/4 of avocado, sliced thinly

1 slice of beef tomato

2 slices of Ezekiel bread

CHEESE, FRUIT AND SPINACH MELTS

Low calorie yet loaded with protein, you cannot go wrong with this easy to prepare lunch sandwich..

CALORIES PER SERVING: 395

PROTEIN: 22

CARBS: 43

FAT: 15G

SERVES 2

4 slices of Ezekiel bread

1 piece of apple, thinly sliced

100g of grated low fat cheese

2 tsp of mustard

50g of spinach

HOW TO MAKE:

Pre-heat Panini/sandwich press (or non-stick skillet) over a medium heat setting.

Spread mustard lightly and evenly on each bread slice.

Layer the slices of apples, spinach and cheese on 2 bread slices. Top with the remaining 2 slices of bread.

Coat the Panini press (or skillet) with cooking spray, and grill the sandwiches for around 5 minutes or until the bread is toasted and cheese is melted.

Remove from the pan and set aside to cool slightly.

Serve.

SUPER
SPAGHETTI SQUASH

A healthy variation to the popular Italian favourite, it is loaded with protein or muscle building.

CALORIES PER SERVING: 295

PROTEIN: 20G

CARBS: 20G

FAT: 15G

SERVES 4

390g of tempeh , cubed

1 spaghetti squash or pumpkin, halved and deseeded

3 tbsp of tamari or soy sauce

2 tbsp of mirin

1 can of chopped tomatoes

1 tbsp of olive oil

2 cloves of garlic, chopped finely

50g of small broccoli florets

50g of baby spinach

HOW TO MAKE:

Pre-heat the oven to (375°F/190 °C/Gas Mark 5).

Get a medium-sized bowl and toss together the tamari, tempeh, garlic, and mirin. Marinate and set aside for 30 minutes.

Get a large baking dish and arrange the squash halves with the cut sides down. Pour half a cup of water into the dish. Bake for around 45 minutes or until tender. Take the dish out of the oven. Turn the squash over and allow to slightly cool.

Get a large skillet and heat oil at medium heat. Add tempeh and cook for 7 to 8 minutes until golden brown, occasionally stirring. Remove the tempeh and keep warm on a plate.

In a medium-sized pot, heat chopped tomatoes at medium heat, and then add the broccoli and allow to cook until tender (around 5 minutes.) Stir the spinach in and remove from heat.

Use a fork to scrape off spaghetti squash strands onto a platter. Spoon some broccoli and hot chopped tomatoes over the dish. Serve with tempeh on top.

JASON'S QUINOA
& CHICKPEA INFUSION

This is another comfort dish which tastes great!

CALORIES PER SERVING: 305

PROTEIN: 15

CARBS: 50

FAT: 5

SERVES 3

1 can of chickpeas

Handful of diced olives

100g quinoa, rinsed

250g of chopped tomatoes

250ml of vegetable broth

2 pieces of squash, diced

2 cloves of garlic, chopped

½ onion, diced

1 red onion, diced

1 tsp of oregano

1 tsp of basil

1 tsp of thyme

HOW TO MAKE:

Sauté the onion, garlic, and squash in a large-sized saucepan over a medium heat.

Put the tomatoes in to the pan and allow to cook for 5 minutes.

Pour in the broth and boil.

Next, add the quinoa and chickpeas. Cover and lower the heat. Allow to cook for about 10 to 15 minutes or until most of the water is absorbed.

Add the herbs and olives and stir through.

Remove from saucepan and serve.

MUSCLE
MILLET & QUINOA

A light dish just right for a relaxing rest day or a day off from muscle building workouts..

CALORIES PER SERVING: 409

PROTEIN: 11G

CARBS: 80G

FAT: 5G

SERVES 2

120g of millet

120g of quinoa

1 diced banana

½ liter of almond milk

½ liter of water

½ tsp of ground ginger

½ cinnamon stick

2 pieces of star anise

2 pieces of cardamom pods

1 tsp of honey

HOW TO MAKE:

Use a sieve to rinse the millet and quinoa under cold running water.

Tip into the crockpot.

Boil water in a pan over a high heat and add the spices and almond milk.

Pour everything into the crockpot.

Put the lid on and set heat to low. Cook for 8 to 9 hours or overnight.

The porridge dish should be creamy and rich when done.

Ladle into bowls and pour over some honey for a treat.

Serve with diced banana.

TITAN
CHILI TOFU

This is a great tasting tofu dish that is easy to prepare; ideal for when you like to spice things up a bit!

CALORIES PER SERVING: 329

PROTEIN: 30

CARBS: 10

FAT: 19

SERVES 1

225g of extra-firm tofu, drained, divided into 4 pieces

1 tbsp of rice vinegar

1 tbsp of soy sauce

½ tsp of hot chili sauce

½ tsp of ginger, minced

A pinch of salt and black pepper

HOW TO MAKE:

Combine vinegar, soy sauce, chilli sauce, and ginger in a small bowl.

Sprinkle the tofu with salt & pepper.

Heat a non-stick skillet over a medium heat. Cook the tofu until browned on both sides, or 3 minutes for each side.

Add the soy sauce mixture and cook for half a minute, constantly stirring.

Transfer to serving dish.

BRAWNY
TOFU STEAKS

For the new vegetarian bodybuilder who is new to tofu dishes, this is one good way to introduce this vegetarian ingredient.

CALORIES PER SERVING: 315

PROTEIN: 30

CARBS: 15

FAT: 15

SERVES 2

240g of extra firm tofu

2 tsp of garlic powder

2 tsp of coriander, ground

2 tsp of chilli powder

½ cup of tamari

HOW TO MAKE:

Cut the tofu into slices.

Combine all other ingredients in one bowl. Pour the mixture over the slices.

Allow to marinate for an hour, store in the refrigerator in a sealed container.

Fry in a little olive oil over a medium heat for 7-8 minutes.

Serve with cooked rice or noodles.

BRAWNY
BARLEY & QUINOA CASSEROLE

Barley is high in fibre and protein and this is a great warm dish to fuel you through your workouts.

CALORIES PER SERVING: 587

PROTEIN: 28G

CARBS: 31G

FAT: 39G

SERVES 6

100g of barley

100g of cooked quinoa

1 green chilli, finely chopped

3 cups of water

200g cheddar cheese, shredded

150g of sour cream

HOW TO MAKE:

Get a lidded saucepan and boil water over a high heat.

Add the barley, and continue to boil. Set heat to low. Cook with lid on for around 45 minutes or until the liquid is significantly absorbed and the barley is tender. Take off the heat and allow to cool slightly.

Mix barley with the shredded cheese, quinoa, chillies, and sour cream in a large-sized bowl.

Serve and enjoy.

SIDES

Side dishes include appetizers, soups, salads, and dips that are served before or together with the main course. For vegetarians, these dishes are important as they complement the entree and complete a vegetarian bodybuilder's dietary requirements, specifically for protein.

BRAWNY GUACAMOLE HUMMUS

Guacamole and houmous in one bowl – both tasty and healthy!

CALORIES PER SERVING: 250

PROTEIN: 10G

CARBS: 30G

FAT: 10G

HOW TO MAKE:

Process all the ingredients in a blender or food processor.

Transfer to a serving dish.

SERVES 3

1 can of chickpeas

1 avocado, chopped finely

1 jalapeno chopped finely

½ tsp of tabasco

1 tbsp of tahini

20g of cilantro, chopped

1 lime, juiced

MUSCLE RANCH HUMMUS

Try this healthy hummus with a bit of American twist; just as healthy, and tastes just as good.

CALORIES PER SERVING: 130

PROTEIN: 10G

CARBS: 19G

FAT: 1

HOW TO MAKE:

Process all the ingredients in a blender or food processor.

Transfer to a serving dish.

SERVES 4

1 can of chickpeas

1 tsp of dried parsley

1 tsp of dried dill

1/3 jar of tahini

1 garlic clove

5 tbsp of Greek yogurt

LEAN
POTATO SALAD

This is an ordinary American side dish that is made healthier in this recipe.

CALORIES PER SERVING: 192

PROTEIN: 9G

CARBS: 30G

FAT: 4G

SERVES 4

450g of small white potatoes, cut into pieces

225g of low-fat plain yogurt

2 tbsp of Dijon mustard

¼ red onion, chopped finely

Pinch of salt and pepper to taste

HOW TO MAKE:

Boil water in a large pot on a high heat.

Cook the potatoes until tender.

Set aside after draining to cool down.

Combine Dijon mustard, plain yogurt, seasoning and red onion in a big bowl.

Add the cooled potatoes. Mix well.

Allow to chill in the refrigerator for at least 2 hours.

Take out of the fridge when ready to serve. Enjoy!

SUPER
GUACAMOLE & RED ONION QUINOA

Healthy and tasty!

CALORIES PER SERVING: 329

PROTEIN: 9

CARBS: 44

FAT: 28

HOW TO MAKE:

Get a mixing bowl and toss in the quinoa, avocado, tomato, red onion, and cilantro. Add lime and other spices to taste.

Refrigerate. Best served cold.

SERVES 1

1 diced avocado

125g of cooked quinoa

1 beef tomato, chopped

1/4 red onion, chopped

1 wedge of lime

2 tbsp of fresh coriander (cilantro), chopped

1 tsp of salt

1 tsp of black pepper

1 tsp of cumin

WALNUT & BLUEBERRY QUINOA

A nutrient-packed side dish!

CALORIES PER SERVING: 593

PROTEIN: 16

CARBS: 84

FAT: 23

HOW TO MAKE:

Mix everything well using a spoon.

SERVES 1

75g of cooked Quinoa

50g of walnuts

50g of blueberries

1 tsp cinnamon

2 tsp of honey

KALE
DIP

This vegetarian dip is creamy and delicious – but with a lot less fat than your average dip on the side.

CALORIES PER SERVING: 30

PROTEIN: 4

CARBS: 6

FAT: 2

SERVES 10

1 bunch of kale

25g of spinach

1 small onion, diced finely

¼ cup of water

2 cloves of garlic, minced

75g of low-fat Greek yogurt

2 tbsp of low-fat mayonnaise

Juice of 1 lemon

Pinch of salt & pepper

HOW TO MAKE:

Heat water, onions, kale, spinach and garlic in a large-sized saucepan over a high heat.

Set the heat to medium, cover and allow to cook for about 15 minutes until the water has evaporated and the kale is tender.

Place the mixture in a food processor and puree.

Get another bowl and stir the yogurt, mayonnaise, onion and lemon juice together.

Add the veggie puree once cool.

Stir some more while adding a dash of salt & pepper to taste.

Immediately serve.

GOURMET GREEN BEANS

You can enjoy a hearty Thanksgiving dinner without fear of jeopardizing your muscle-building goals. This side dish will allow you to indulge and is packed with vitamins and iron!

CALORIES PER SERVING: 270

PROTEIN: 4G

CARBS: 15G

FAT: 2G

SERVES 4

400g green beans

2 tsp of olive oil

1 red pepper, cut into strips

1 yellow pepper, cut into strips

½ tsp of red pepper, flaked

1 clove of garlic, finely chopped

1 tsp of sesame oil

½ tsp of salt

¼ tsp of black pepper, freshly ground

½ tsp of onion powder

HOW TO MAKE:

Drop the beans in a saucepan of boiling water.

Allow to cook for about 3 minutes or until the desired tenderness is achieved.

Drain the beans and put in cold water to prevent further cooking.

Get a new saucepan and fry peppers lightly in olive oil at medium heat.

Once softened, add green beans, garlic, red pepper flakes, salt & pepper, onion powder, and sesame oil.

Once spices are distributed evenly, transfer to a serving dish.

Serve hot.

BRAWNY
BLACK BEAN & SWEET POTATO SIDE

Protein-packed side dish that brings a lot of flavour – especially if you love chilli!

CALORIES PER SERVING: 238

PROTEIN: 15G

CARBS: 40

FAT: 2

SERVES 2

150g of black beans	1 piece of small onion, diced	½ tsp of garlic powder
150g of cannellini beans	½ piece of red bell pepper, chopped	2 tbsp of olive oil
2 sweet potatoes, peeled & chopped		1 tsp of cumin
2 pieces of medium carrots, sliced	400g of chopped tomatoes	½ tsp of cayenne
	50ml of vegetable broth	½ tsp of salt
2 cloves of garlic, minced	1 tbsp of chili powder	¼ tsp of black pepper

HOW TO MAKE:

Heat olive oil in a pan over a medium heat.

Sautee garlic and onions for about 1 or 2 minutes.

Add carrots, bell pepper, and sweet potatoes for about 6 minutes or until the onions are soft.

Lower heat setting to medium-low, then add the rest of the ingredients. Stir to mix well.

Cover partially and simmer.

Allow to cook for around 25 minutes, occasionally stirring until veggies are cooked, and the flavours have blended well.

Serve.

SWEET
POTATO & GREEN PEA SOUP

Fat-free and completely vegan recipe – just for the taste of curry!

CALORIES PER SERVING: 173

PROTEIN: 6G

CARBS: 35G

FAT: 1G

SERVES 2

280g of green split peas, dried

1 large carrot, chopped

2 small sweet potatoes, chopped

1 stalk of celery, chopped

5 cups of water

½ onion, chopped

½ tsp of garlic powder

½ piece of bay leaf

½ tsp of dried oregano

½ tsp of curry powder

¼ tsp of pepper

¼ tsp of salt

HOW TO MAKE:

Combine water, split peas, onion, and other spices in a large-sized sauce pan on a medium to low heat.

Allow to simmer uncovered for about 1 hour.

Add the rest of the ingredients. Continue to simmer, this time covered, for 45 minutes more or just until the desired soup thickness is reached. Stir occasionally.

Remove the bay leaf.

Transfer everything into a blender, and process.

Reheat slightly before serving.

MUSCLE
LENTIL SOUP

You will definitely enjoy the perfect blend of spices in this very traditional warming soup! Lentils are packed with protein and goodness.

CALORIES PER SERVING: 398

PROTEIN: 25G

CARBS: 70G

FAT: 2G

SERVES 2

200ml of vegetable broth

1 tsp of olive oil

1 carrot, sliced

150g of brown lentils

1 onion, diced

2 tsp of lemon juice

2 bay leaves

Salt & pepper, to taste

¼ tsp of dried thyme

HOW TO MAKE:

Sauté carrot and onion in sunflower oil on a medium heat for around 5 minutes or until onions have become translucent.

Add lentils, bay leaves, thyme, salt & pepper, and vegetable broth. Lower heat and simmer. Put the lid on and allow to cook for about 40 to 45 minutes, just to make sure the lentils have softened.

Take the leaves out, and stir the lemon juice in.

Serve hot.

BRAWNY BLACK BEAN SOUP

This is a tasty and easy to prepare bean soup that can get you all warmed up and ready to power on in only 15 minutes!

CALORIES PER SERVING: 231

PROTEIN: 18

CARBS: 42

FAT: 5

HOW TO MAKE:

Pulse half of the beans in food processor with a bit of water until smooth.

Put all beans in a medium-sized saucepan. Add salsa, chilli powder, and vegetable broth. Bring to a boil on a high heat. Top with cheese and onions.

Serve and enjoy!

SERVES 4

800g of black beans, undrained

450ml of vegetable broth

50g of salsa

2 tbsp of chili powder

2 tbsp of garlic powder

50g of cheddar cheese, shredded

1 chopped red onion

A pinch of salt and pepper

PROTEIN
PACKED EGG & BEAN SALAD

A classic American favorite dish cooked with three kinds of beans. It is nutrient-packed as well!

CALORIES PER SERVING: 366

PROTEIN: 15G

CARBS: 30G

FAT: 14G

SERVES 8

420g of cooked black beans, drained & rinsed

420g of cooked cannellini beans, drained & rinsed

420g of cooked kidney beans, drained & rinsed

6 hard-boiled eggs, sliced

1 celery stick chopped

½ onion, chopped

20g olives, sliced

3 tsp of hot pepper sauce

½ tsp of salt

¼ tsp of pepper

3 tsp of Italian salad dressing e

HOW TO MAKE:

Drain the beans, then rinse, and finally drain again.

Combine celery, olives, onions, salad dressing, seasonings, and beans.

Carefully mix. Refrigerate for at least 2 hours, preferably overnight.

When ready to serve. Drain off the salad dressing first, then add vegetarian mayo and eggs.

Carefully mix so as not to mash the beans.

Serve.

BULGUR WHEAT, FETA CHEESE & QUINOA SALAD

A variation of the traditional tabbouleh salad, this version features feta cheese that provides for a tasty twist, without compromising on nutrients.

CALORIES PER SERVING: 350

PROTEIN: 15G

CARBS: 50G

FAT: 15G

HOW TO MAKE:

Mix bulgur wheat with boiling water in a large-sized bowl. Cover and set aside for half an hour before draining.

Add lemon juice and pesto. Stir using a whisk.

Combine pesto mixture, bulgur, quinoa, feta, tomatoes, green onions, chickpeas, pepper, parsley in a large bowl. Gently toss to mix well.

Serve.

SERVES 4

75g of bulgur wheat, uncooked

75g of cooked quinoa

420g of chickpeas, drained

75g of feta cheese, crumbled

200g cherry tomatoes, chopped

½ jar of pesto

3 tbsp of fresh lemon juice

2 tbsp of fresh parsley, minced

1/4 tsp of black pepper

1 onion, sliced thinly

2 cups of water, boiling

SNACKS

A healthy snack is important because it provides you with a great opportunity to supplement your nutrient intake, without getting you side-tracked from your fitness goals. It also relieves hunger pangs that you feel in between regular meals. Following are healthy snacks that can help boost your muscle building efforts.

PROTEIN PACKED
GREEK YOGURT WITH HONEY & ALMONDS

Nutritious and healthy, this snack is sure to quell your mid-afternoon hunger pangs and provide an instant energy boost!

CALORIES PER SERVING: 451

PROTEIN: 44G

CARBS: 33G

FAT: 19G

HOW TO MAKE:

Just mix all the ingredients together, and start snacking. Enjoy!

SERVES 1

225g of Greek yogurt

1 scoop of Vanilla protein powder

30g of roasted almonds

1 tsp of honey, to sweeten

POWER
ALMOND BUTTER HUMMUS

If you haven't tried this dish yet, you may think that an almond butter-houmous combo would result in something gross. You'll be surprised that this recipe is actually really appetizing and quite healthy, too!

CALORIES PER SERVING: 308

PROTEIN: 19G

CARBS: 27

FAT: 16G

HOW TO MAKE:

Combine all ingredients in a blender and process.

Transfer to serving bowl.

SERVES 4

50g of crunchy almond butter

1 can of chickpeas, drained

2 tbsp of olive oil

½ piece of lemon (juice only)

1 garlic clove

MUSCLE
FETA CHEESE & OLIVES

This is a quick and easy snack to prepare mid-afternoon instead of stuffing yourself with cake.

CALORIES PER SERVING: 305

PROTEIN: 24G

CARBS: 9G

FAT: 18G

HOW TO MAKE:

Cut feta cheese into small cubes. Pair each cube with a kalamata olive on a cocktail stick.

Enjoy your refreshing snack!

SERVES 1

110g of feta cheese

10 kalamata olives

Cocktail sticks

QUICK FIX
ROASTED BEANS

Great for that sudden mid-afternoon craving while at the same time giving you a quick protein fix.

CALORIES PER SERVING: 336

PROTEIN: 21

CARBS: 51

FAT: 6

SERVES 1

1 can of garbanzo beans

HOW TO MAKE:

Preheat oven (375°F/190 °C/Gas Mark 5).

Open a 15-oz can of garbanzo beans; drain and rinse the contents, then pat dry.

Roast for around 30 to 40 minutes or just after the beans turn brown and crispy.

Sprinkle with some salt. Your snack is ready.

SUPER
SWEET POTATO FRIES

This is the high quality version of the fast-food staple French fries – but much healthier and less greasy!

CALORIES PER SERVING: 162

PROTEIN: 2G

CARBS: 25G

FAT: 7G

SERVES 4

2 large sweet potatoes, cut into thin strips

1 tsp of cumin

1 tbsp of olive oil

½ tsp of seasoned salt

¼ tsp of paprika

1 dash of cayenne pepper

HOW TO MAKE:

Preheat oven (375°F/190 °C/Gas Mark 5).

Put the sweet potato strips into a large bowl.

Drizzle with some olive oil. Sprinkle the rest of the ingredients over the top.

Toss together gently to evenly and fully coat the potatoes.

Get a baking sheet and arrange the coated potatoes in 1 layer. Bake for around 30 minutes.

Allow to cool down for a few minutes.

Serve.

PERFECT HUMMUS

An all-time Mediterranean classic, the time-tested fresh and light flavour of its simple ingredients is a sure-fire hit!

CALORIES PER SERVING: 280

PROTEIN: 11G

CARBS: 23G

FAT: 17G

HOW TO MAKE:

Combine all ingredients in a blender and process.

Transfer to serving bowl.

SERVES 4

1 can of chickpeas

1/3 jar of tahini

3 tbsp of olive oil

1 lemon (juice only)

1 garlic clove

Pinch of salt and pepper

PROTEIN PACKED LATTE

A cup of this smooth, protein rich tea latte is sure to drive any cold winter night woes away, and make any evening special.

CALORIES PER SERVING: 206

PROTEIN: 30G

CARBS: 16G

FAT: 1G

HOW TO MAKE:

Boil water and pour into a mug. Add chai spice mix, stevia and protein powder.

Stir until everything is blended well.

Serve immediately. Sip and enjoy the latte goodness!

SERVES 1

1 scoop of vanilla protein powder

1 packet of stevia

1 tsp of chai spice mix (decaf)

POWER
EGGPLANT GANOUSH

Similar to hummus, ganoush is a Middle Eastern snack/dip, but made with eggplant.

CALORIES PER SERVING: 275

PROTEIN: 7G

CARBS: 28G

FAT: 15G

SERVES 2

1 medium-sized aubergine (egg-plant)

1 can of garbanzo beans, drained

1 clove of garlic

1 tbsp tahini

A pinch of sea salt

1 large lemon (juice only)

2 tsp of olive oil

1 tbsp of fresh parsley, chopped

HOW TO MAKE:

Divide the eggplant into 2.

Preheat oven (400°F/200 °C/Gas Mark 6).

Roast for about 45 minutes or until soft.

Set aside to cool slightly. Scoop out the inside of the aubergine, leaving only the skin.

Mix with the rest of the ingredients (except for the oil and parsley) and process in a blender until a smooth consistency is achieved.

Add olive oil and process until blended into a smooth pulp.

Mix the parsley in to serve.

VANILLA PROTEIN
GREEK YOGURT & BLACKBERRIES

Enjoy the taste of the high-protein yogurt, and get an instant hunger pang relief.

CALORIES PER SERVING: 206

PROTEIN: 37G

CARBS: 16

FAT: 5

HOW TO MAKE:

Add all of the ingredients into a serving bowl.

Enjoy your snack!

SERVES 1

170g of Greek Yogurt

1 scoop of vanilla protein powder

75g of blackberries

75g of blueberries

OVEN-ROASTED CHICKPEAS

Low-fat and high in protein, this nut makes a great mid-day snack.

CALORIES PER SERVING: 193

PROTEIN: 10

CARBS: 30

FAT: 7

SERVES 2

340g of chickpeas , drained and rinsed

1 tbsp of olive oil

1 tsp of garlic powder

½ tsp of salt

½ tsp of pepper

HOW TO MAKE:

Preheat oven (350°F/180 °C/Gas Mark 4).

Pat chickpeas to dry, then coat well with oil by tossing gently.

Get a baking tray, and arrange the chickpeas in 1 layer. Sprinkle with salt and garlic powder.

Roast for about 40 minutes (or until crispy) shaking one or two times to turn.

Serve.

HOMEMADE PROTEIN SHAKES

If you want to spend hundreds of pounds on pre-made shakes full of chemicals and fillers that cements onto your kitchen sink then be my guest! If not, try these homemade healthy alternatives that will pack on just as much punch as the shop-bought varieties.

GREEN & MEAN

Begin your day with this easy to prepare veggie-rich breakfast that packs a monstrous protein-powered punch. Go Green!

CALORIES PER SERVING: 497

PROTEIN: 28

CARBS: 62

FAT: 17

HOW TO MAKE:

Place all the ingredients together in the blender and process until the desired consistency is achieved.

Pour contents of the blender into a tall glass. Serve immediately and enjoy!

SERVES 1

3 stalks of Celery

3 bunches of Kale

½ cup of sliced pineapple

½ apple, chopped

A handful of spinach

1 tbsp of coconut oil

1 scoop of vanilla protein powder

CHOCOLATE PEANUT DELIGHT

Get your chocolate fix with this tasty shake.

CALORIES PER SERVING: 656

PROTEIN: 63G

CARBS: 55G

FAT: 21G

HOW TO MAKE:

Add all the ingredients to a blender and blend until smooth.

Enjoy!

SERVES 1

1 scoop of chocolate whey protein powder

1 cup of low-fat Greek yogurt

1 whole banana

2 tbsp of peanut butter

1 cup of ice

JASON'S
HOMEMADE MASS GAINER

It can be hard to get in the necessary calories to grow. Most weight gainers contain empty calories and can be expensive. This beast of a shake contains around 1000 healthy calories and a whopping 75g of Protein to keep you growing.

CALORIES PER SERVING: 970

PROTEIN: 75G

CARBS: 90G

FAT: 30G

HOW TO MAKE:

Add all the ingredients to a blender and blend until smooth.

Enjoy!

SERVES 1

2 scoop of chocolate whey protein powder

500ml of whole milk

55g of dry rolled oats

1 whole banana

2 tbsp of organic almond butter

1 cup of crushed ice

BERRY
PROTEIN SHAKE

Totally refreshing on a hot summer's day and it works well any time of the year.

CALORIES PER SERVING: 342

PROTEIN: 38G

CARBS: 42G

FAT: 3G

HOW TO MAKE:

Add all the ingredients to a blender and blend until smooth.

Enjoy!

SERVES 1

2 scoop of whey protein powder

1 cup of blueberries

1 cup of blackberries

1 cup of raspberries

1 cup of water

1 cup of ice

FRESH STRAWBERRY SHAKE

Keep it simple with this strawberry shake all year round

CALORIES PER SERVING: 303

PROTEIN: 35G

CARBS: 15G

FAT: 11G

HOW TO MAKE:

Add all the ingredients to a blender and blend until smooth.

Enjoy!

SERVES 1

2 scoops of vanilla protein powder

1 cup of strawberries

2 cups of water

1 tbsp of flaxseed oil

CHOCO
COFFEE ENERGY SHAKE

Swap your average morning caffeine hit with this refreshing alternative.

CALORIES PER SERVING: 299

PROTEIN: 42G

CARBS: 14G

FAT: 6G

HOW TO MAKE:

Add all the ingredients to a blender and blend until smooth.

Enjoy!

SERVES 1

2 scoops of chocolate protein powder

100ml of low-fat milk

1 cup of water

1 tbsp of instant coffee

LEAN AND MEAN
PINEAPPLE SHAKE

Fresh, tropical and zingy – this shake really packs a punch and is crammed full with energy to keep you going until at least lunch -time.

CALORIES PER SERVING: 355

PROTEIN: 23G

CARBS: 65G

FAT: 3G

HOW TO MAKE:

Add all the ingredients to a blender and blend until smooth.

Enjoy!

SERVES 1

1 cup chopped pineapple

4 strawberries

1 banana

1 tbsp low-fat Greek yogurt

1 scoop of vanilla protein powder

1 cup of water

CHOPPED ALMOND SMOOTHIE

Quick and easy shake that will ease your chocolate craving and provide you with 24 grams of protein.

CALORIES PER SERVING: 241

PROTEIN: 24G

CARBS: 6G

FAT: 13G

HOW TO MAKE:

Add all the ingredients to a blender and blend until smooth.

Enjoy!

SERVES 1

1 1/2 cups water

17 chopped almonds

1/2 tsp coconut extract

1 scoop chocolate protein powder

VANILLA
STRAWBERRY SURPRISE

If this doesn't transport you back to a day out by the seaside nothing will – it tastes amazing and is deceptively good at filling you up and helping you to bulk up and shred fat.

CALORIES PER SERVING: 329

PROTEIN: 36G

CARBS: 42G

FAT: 2G

HOW TO MAKE:

Add all the ingredients to a blender and blend until smooth.

Enjoy!

SERVES 1

2 scoops of vanilla protein powder

1 cup of ice

1 banana

4 fresh or frozen strawberries

BREAKFAST
BANANA SHAKE

Not much time? This breakfast shake packs a punch and will ensure a positive start to your day

CALORIES PER SERVING: 566

PROTEIN: 59G

CARBS: 69G

FAT: 6G

HOW TO MAKE:

Add all the ingredients to a blender and blend until smooth.

Enjoy!

SERVES 1

200ml low-fat milk

1 banana

100g of rolled oats

2 scoops of vanilla whey protein powder

PEACHY PUNCH

This peachy punch will satisfy your sweet tooth as well as providing 50 grams of protein.

CALORIES PER SERVING: 543

PROTEIN: 50G

CARBS: 57G

FAT: 11G

HOW TO MAKE:

Add all the ingredients to a blender and blend until smooth.

Enjoy!

SERVES 1

2 scoop of vanilla protein powder

200ml of low-fat milk

45g of rolled oats

1 chopped peach

1 cup of water

50g of low fat Greek yogurt

BLACKBERRY BRAWN

Quick and easy shake that is as tasty as it is nutritious.

CALORIES PER SERVING: 457

PROTEIN: 47G

CARBS: 30G

FAT: 16G

HOW TO MAKE:

Add all the ingredients to a blender and blend until smooth.

Enjoy!

SERVES 1

1 cup of blackberries

200ml of low–fat milk

2 tbsp of Flax Seed oil

50g of low-fat Greek yogurt

2 scoops of vanilla protein powder

1 Cup Ice

NO
WHEY!

No protein powder? This healthy, tasty shake contains a nice dose of protein to keep you growing!

CALORIES PER SERVING: 388

PROTEIN: 26G

CARBS: 32G

FAT: 22G

HOW TO MAKE:

Add all the ingredients to a blender and blend until smooth.

Enjoy!

SERVES 1

1 cup of blackberries

1 cup of strawberries

200ml of low–fat milk

130g of Greek yogurt

1 tbsp of almond butter

1 cup Ice

CARIBBEAN CRUSH

Absolutely delicious!

CALORIES PER SERVING: 263

PROTEIN: 25G

CARBS: 38G

FAT: 3G

HOW TO MAKE:

Add all the ingredients to a blender and blend until smooth.

Enjoy!

SERVES 1

1 scoop of protein powder (your choice)

½ chopped mango

½ cup of pineapple chunks

1 peeled and cubed kiwi

1 strawberry

1 cup of ice cubes

CHOCOLATE & RASPBERRY BANG

A tasty, quick protein shake to keep you growing and shredding!

CALORIES PER SERVING: 269

PROTEIN: 31G

CARBS: 16G

FAT: 9G

HOW TO MAKE:

Add all the ingredients to a blender and blend until smooth.

Enjoy!

SERVES 1

2 scoops of chocolate protein powder

1/2 cup of raspberries

200ml of whole milk

1/2 cup of ice cubes

CINNAMON SURPRISE

Quick and easy protein shake to satisfy your taste buds!

CALORIES PER SERVING: 244

PROTEIN: 47G

CARBS: 7G

FAT: 4G

HOW TO MAKE:

Add all the ingredients to a blender and blend until smooth.

Enjoy!

SERVES 1

2 scoops of chocolate protein powder

1 tbsp of cinnamon

1 cup of water

1 cup of ice

PUMPKIN POWER

A great tasting shake that's packed full of protein.

CALORIES PER SERVING: 224

PROTEIN: 38G

CARBS: 14G

FAT: 3G

HOW TO MAKE:

Add all the ingredients to a blender and blend until smooth.

Enjoy!

SERVES 1

2 scoops of vanilla protein powder

1 cup of chopped pumpkin

1 tsp cinnamon

1 cup of water

LIME
POWER SHAKE

Bursting with Vitamin C goodness, this power shake is packed with muscle building protein as well!

CALORIES PER SERVING: 350

PROTEIN: 32G

CARBS: 52G

FAT: 6G

HOW TO MAKE:

Combine almond milk, protein powder, key lime juice, maple syrup, banana, and ice in the blender and process until smooth. Top the shake with graham cracker crumbs and a dollop of yogurt.

Serve in a tall glass!

SERVES 1

2 scoops of vanilla protein powder

1 piece of banana

1 cup of almond milk, unsweetened

1 tbsp of key lime juice

1 key lime zest

1 tbsp of non-fat Greek yogurt

1 tbsp of crushed graham crackers

1 cup of ice cubes

½ tsp of maple syrup

DESSERTS

Just because you are trying to build muscles doesn't mean you cannot indulge in sweet goodies once in a while. There are vegetarian desserts that are not only healthy, but rich in protein as well. Thus, your fitness goals will not be compromised. Here are some dessert recipes that you can try.

CHOCOLATE & PEANUT PUDDING PIE

A simple and easy recipe to make, this mouth-watering dessert is both cool and creamy. Even more, it is packed with a lot of muscle-boosting protein.

CALORIES PER SERVING: 322

PROTEIN: 20G

CARBS: 20G

FAT: 18G

SERVES 1

1 pack of zero-fat, sugar-free chocolate pudding

250ml of not-fat milk

2 scoops of chocolate-flavored protein powder

3 tbsp of crunchy peanut butter

Handful of roasted walnuts

85g of whipped cream

1 piece of chocolate pie crust

HOW TO MAKE:

Mix the protein powder with pudding powder.

Stir the whipped cream and milk in until the mixture thickens.

Pour the mixture into the piecrust; allow it to cool in the refrigerator for half an hour.

Garnish with the peanut butter and walnuts. Serve and enjoy!

JASON'S
PEANUT PROTEIN BARS

Save your money with these delicious, homemade protein bars!

CALORIES PER BAR: 386

PROTEIN: 18G

CARBS: 24G

FAT: 6G

MAKES 12 BARS

4 scoops of vanilla protein powder

400g of rolled oats

340g of almond butter

250ml of coconut cream

HOW TO MAKE:

Get a bowl and add the coconut cream and whisk until smooth, then add the protein powder and peanut butter and mix thoroughly.

Pour the oats into the bowl and again mix through.

Scoop out the mixture into a baking tray and flatten until the surface is smooth.

Place the tray in the fridge and leave for around 8 hours.

Cut into 12 bars.

POWER
PARFAIT

A delicious dessert that tastes a great as it looks. Contains a whopping 38g of protein.

CALORIES PER SERVING: 254

PROTEIN: 38G

CARBS: 21G

FAT: 2G

HOW TO MAKE:

Mix the yogurt with the protein powder.

Get a tall parfait glass and layer with berries and yogurt.

SERVES 1

1 scoop of vanilla protein powder

2 cups of mixed berries

200ml of Greek yogurt

STRAWBERRY
AND BANANA PROTEIN PUDDING

This is definitely a better alternative to yogurt-coated raisins. Though this simple recipe only has a few ingredients, it is not lacking in flavour and nutrients!

CALORIES PER SERVING: 195

PROTEIN: 23G

CARBS: 13G

FAT: 7G

SERVES 1

1 scoop of strawberry protein powder

60ml of egg whites

1 tbsp, non-fat, sugar-free chocolate pudding

3 pieces of strawberries, sliced

1 piece of small banana, sliced

Handful of blueberries

2 tbsp of water

HOW TO MAKE:

Combine the pudding and protein powder.

Add water and egg whites; mix well to achieve thick consistency.

Add powder if texture is still runny.

Spoon the batter out and transfer to a small plate.

Put in the freezer for half an hour.

Garnish with the strawberries, banana and blueberries

POWER
PROTEIN WAFFLES

Who said waffles were unhealthy? Never mind, these are a great alternative

CALORIES PER SERVING: 314

PROTEIN: 37G

CARBS: 28G

FAT: 5G

HOW TO MAKE:

Add all the ingredients into a blender and blend.

Add the mixture to a waffle iron and bake.

SERVES 1

4 eggs whites

1 scoop of vanilla protein powder

40g of rolled oats

1 tsp of baking powder

½ tsp of stevia

BRAWNY BANANA PROTEIN COOKIES

This recipe is a must try recipe for banana lovers.

CALORIES PER SERVING: 359

PROTEIN: 25G

CARBS: 40G

FAT: 11G

SERVES 2

2 bananas

110g of oatmeal

2 scoop of vanilla protein powder

2 tsp of cinnamon

¼ tsp of baking powder

Handful of finely chopped walnuts or almonds

HOW TO MAKE:

Pre-heat the oven to 180C/350F/Gas Mark 4.

Oil-spray a non-stick pan.

Lightly oil-spray a cookie sheet. Distribute the oil evenly using a paper towel.

Get a large-sized bowl and mash the bananas until a creamy texture is achieved.

Add protein powder, oat, salt, walnuts, baking powder, and cinnamon. Mix well. Spoon mixture onto cookie sheet, forming cookie shaped pieces.

Bake for around 15 minutes.

Serve.

GREEK YOGURT
WITH HONEY AND BERRIES

A quick and easy dessert that contains a whopping 43g of protein. .

CALORIES PER SERVING: 522

PROTEIN: 43G

CARBS: 86G

FAT: 7G

HOW TO MAKE:

Mix all your ingredients and you've got a fresh and healthy dessert with nothing on your conscience. You could sprinkle flaked almonds over the top for a bit of crunch.

SERVES 1

1 scoop of vanilla protein powder

100g Greek Yoghurt

4 tbsp of honey

45g of berries

POWER
PEANUT CHOCOLATE PANCAKES

Quick and easy great recipe. Contains lots of protein to keep you anabolic and is also low on carbs.

CALORIES PER SERVING: 286

PROTEIN: 33G

CARBS: 16G

FAT: 10G

HOW TO MAKE:

Get a bowl and combine all ingredients. Mix well until you get a thick batter.

Pour the butter on a greased skillet like you would a pancake, frying over a medium heat.

Serve when done cooking.

SERVES 2

1 scoop of chocolate protein powder

1 tbsp of smooth peanut butter

2 egg whites

2 tbsp of raw coconut flour

STRENGTH STRAWBERRY & CHEESE SURPRISE

Another heavenly combination – blueberry and cheese – this is a must-try vegetarian version, especially for muscle builders

CALORIES PER SERVING: 167

PROTEIN: 15G

CARBS: 20G

FAT: 3G

SERVES 4

110g of low-fat cottage cheese

80g of whole strawberry, fresh

60ml of egg whites

60ml of skim milk

100g of whole wheat flour

1 packet of stevia

1 ½ tsp of lemon juice

HOW TO MAKE:

Combine the skim milk, flour, and cottage cheese in a mixing bowl.

Beat the egg whites to get frothy consistency. Add to cheese mixture.

Stir in lemon juice. Toss in the strawberries. Stir again.

Transfer the batter into a non-stick frying pan. Turn when the tops start to bubble, and the bottom part starts to turn brown.

Serve.

PROTEIN
PUMPKIN COOKIES

Caving for cookies? This easy low-fat recipe is sure to give you a healthy fix.

CALORIES PER SERVING: 136

PROTEIN: 10G

CARBS: 15G

FAT: 4G

SERVES 4

2 scoops of vanilla protein powder

2 boxes of spice cake mix

150g of chocolate chips

700g of pumpkin (1 can)

HOW TO MAKE:

Pre-heat the oven to 180C/350F/Gas Mark 4.

Oil-spray a non-stick pan.

Lightly oil-spray a cookie sheet. Distribute the oil evenly using a paper towel.

Get a large-sized bowl and mash the bananas until a creamy texture is achieved.

Add protein powder, oat, salt, walnuts, baking powder, and cinnamon. Mix well. Spoon mixture onto cookie sheet, forming cookie shaped pieces.

Bake for around 15 minutes.

Serve.

COTTAGE CHEESECAKE

A hearty, protein packed cheesecake to enjoy!

CALORIES PER SERVING: 487

PROTEIN: 43G

CARBS: 53G

FAT: 7G

HOW TO MAKE:

Add all the ingredients to a blender and blend until smooth.

Place in a bowl and top with the strawberries.

Place in the fridge for 20 minutes.

SERVES 1

150g of fat free cottage cheese

1 scoop of vanilla protein powder

1 packet of stevia

1 tbsp sugar free instant pudding mix

5 tbsp of low fat milk

Handful of Strawberries

CONVERSION CHARTS

Volume

Imperial	Metric
1 tbsp	15ml
2 fl oz	55 ml
3 fl oz	75 ml
5 fl oz (¼ pint)	150 ml
10 fl oz (½ pint)	275 ml
1 pint	570 ml
1 ¼ pints	725 ml
1 ¾ pints	1 litre
2 pints	1.2 litres
2½ pints	1.5 litres
4 pints	2.25 litres

Weight

Imperial	Metric
½ oz	10 g
¾ oz	20 g
1 oz	25 g
1½ oz	40 g
2 oz	50 g
2½ oz	60 g
3 oz	75 g
4 oz	110 g
4½ oz	125 g
5 oz	150 g
6 oz	175 g
7 oz	200 g
8 oz	225 g
9 oz	250 g
10 oz	275 g
12 oz	350 g
1 lb	450 g
1 lb 8 oz	700 g
2 lb 3 lb	900 g 1.35 kg

Cups	Imperial	Metric
1 cup flour	5oz	150g
1 cup caster or granulated sugar	8oz	225g
1 cup soft brown sugar	6oz	175g
1 cup soft butter/margarine	8oz	225g
1 cup sultanas/raisins	7oz	200g
1 cup currants	5oz	150g
1 cup ground almonds	4oz	110g
1 cup oats	4oz	110g
1 cup golden syrup/honey	12oz	350g
1 cup uncooked rice	7oz	200g
1 cup grated cheese	4oz	110g
1 stick butter	4oz	110g
¼ cup liquid (water, milk, oil etc)	4 tablespoons	60ml
½ cup liquid (water, milk, oil etc)	¼ pint	125ml
1 cup liquid (water, milk, oil etc)	½ pint	250ml

Oven temperatures

Gas Mark	Fahrenheit	Celsius
1/4	225	110
1/2	250	130
1	275	140
2	300	150
3	325	170
4	350	180
5	375	190
6	400	200
7	425	220
8	450	230
9	475	240

BONUS CONTENT:

THE FAST AND FRESH
BODYBUILDING COOKBOOK MEAL PLANS
(100% FREE)

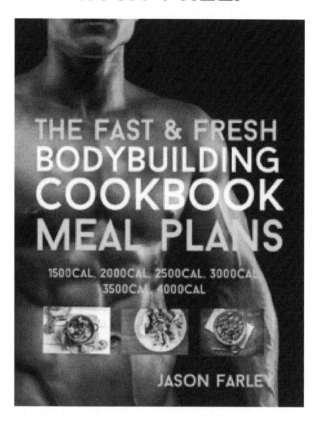

I believe that anyone can build a fantastic body and to ensure you get there, I created
The Fast and Fresh Bodybuilding Cookbook Meal Plans as a counterpart to this cookbook to save you the hard
work when it comes to what to eat, how much to eat and when to eat.

This special manual contains 6 different delicious daily meal plans ranging from 1500 calories all the way to a
whopping 4000 calories, so you're in control of how big or shredded you wanna get!

VISIT : HTTP://BIT.LY/FASTANDFRESHMEALPLANS
TO GET THIS NOW!

WOULD YOU MIND DOING ME A FAVOR?

Thanks again for purchasing my book. I'm confident that you'll love the recipes and hope that they will help you in your quest to burn fat and build more muscle!

Before you leave, I have a little favour to ask. If you enjoyed this book, would you mind taking a minute to write a brief blurb about this book on Amazon? I love to get feedback on my work and I would be really grateful!

OTHER BOOKS
BY ME...

I've been training for over a decade now. Getting in shape can be a hard task with so much misinformation, myths, scams and just plain B.S thrown around in the fitness industry. I see so many people fall for the same false promises every day.

With my books, I want to educate and support you in your quest to achieve all of your fitness goals. Whether you want to build muscle or burn fat and get shredded, there's something here for you. All of my books provide proven, sound training and nutritional advice backed by science (no bro-science here!)

And you won't need a fancy gym membership, tons of money or expensive supplements to be successful with my books - just the desire and willpower to change your life!

I hope you like my books and I look forward to hearing about your amazing transformation!

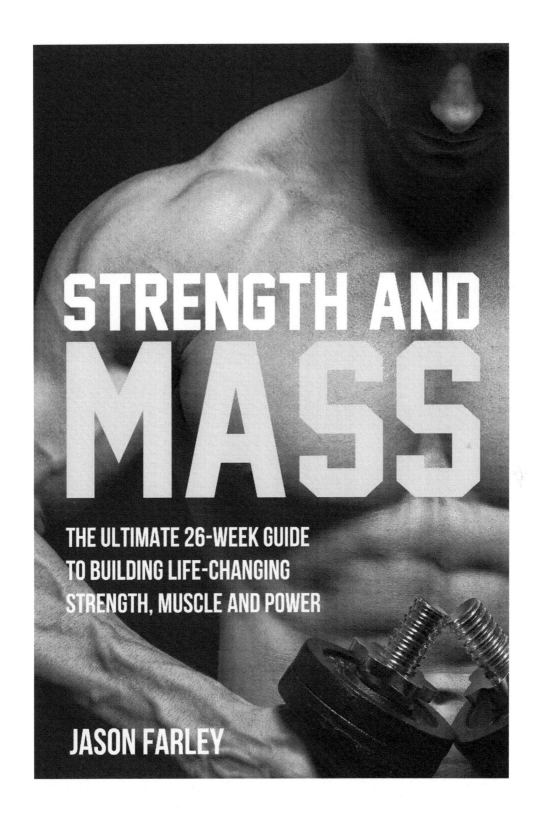

STRENGTH AND MASS

THE ULTIMATE 26-WEEK GUIDE TO BUILDING LIFE-CHANGING STRENGTH, MUSCLE AND POWER

JASON FARLEY

If you want to possess a lean, muscular and strong physique that demands respect and attention wherever you go...without wasting money on worthless supplements or steroids...then STRENGTH AND MASS is your answer.

I'm sure you've wondered what it takes to build a truly unbelievable body. The kind that women love and men envy...

I bet you've asked yourself questions like ...

"What exercises should I be doing?"
"How many days a week should I be training?"
"How many calories should I be eating?"

Well, in this book you're going to learn the answers to these and much, much more.

Strength and Mass is a step-by-step muscle-building program designed to improve size, strength and power without putting on unnecessary body fat. Within these pages, you'll finally learn exactly what it takes to build the body of your dreams.

Strength and Mass includes...

• A comprehensive, detailed and structured 26 week muscle building program – You will be told exactly how many reps, sets and exercises to do and when to do them.
• A fully detailed nutrition guide – You will be given full macronutrient breakdowns and a complete formula for calculating how many calories you need to grow!

And much much more!

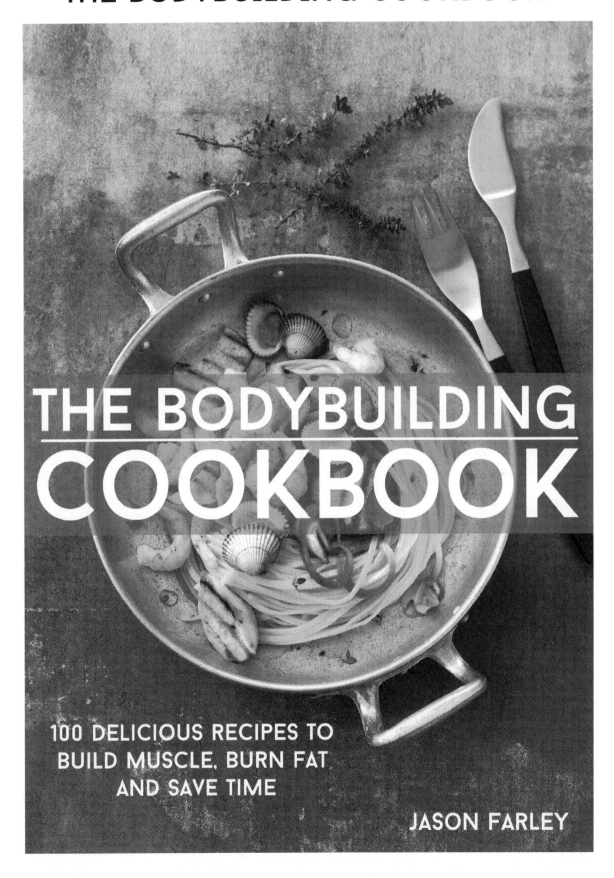

THE BODYBUILDING COOKBOOK

100 DELICIOUS RECIPES TO BUILD MUSCLE, BURN FAT AND SAVE TIME

JASON FARLEY

The Easy Way to Bulk up and Burn Fat Fast!

If you want to learn how to create healthy, delicious and nutritious meals that are specially designed to build muscle, burn fat and save time, then THE BODY-BUILDING COOKBOOK is your answer!

With The Bodybuilding Cookbook, you'll never have to be frustrated with your diet again. You'll learn how to cook healthy, tasty, quick and easy meals that will build quality lean muscle mass, burn fat fast and won't cost you an arm and a leg!

And these recipes aren't just a slight upgrade to familiar bodybuilding meals like you'd find in most health and fitness cookbooks e.g. coating your already bland chicken with some equally bland salsa sauce. These recipes are so delicious your taste buds will believe you're in a 5 star restaurant!

The Bodybuilding Cookbook includes...

* 9 mouth-watering breakfast meals like my Brawny Breakfast Burrito, Banana and Almond Muscle Oatmeal, Power Protein Waffles and Turkey Muscle Omelette. They will kick-start your engine and ensure you start off the day as you mean to go on!

* 18 succulent and delicious chicken and poultry recipes like my Muscle Moroccan Chicken Casserole, Turkey Meatball Fiesta, Anabolic Ratatouille Chicken, Aesthetic Tomato and Olive Pan-Fried Chicken and Chicken Brawn Burger. Say bye bye to boiled bland chicken. These meals will ensure that your body has no choice but to burn fat and build muscle!

* 13 tasty homemade protein shakes like my Chocolate Peanut Delight, Blackberry Brawn, Caribbean Crush, Cinnamon Surprise and my personal delicious Mass Gainer.

* And much, much more...

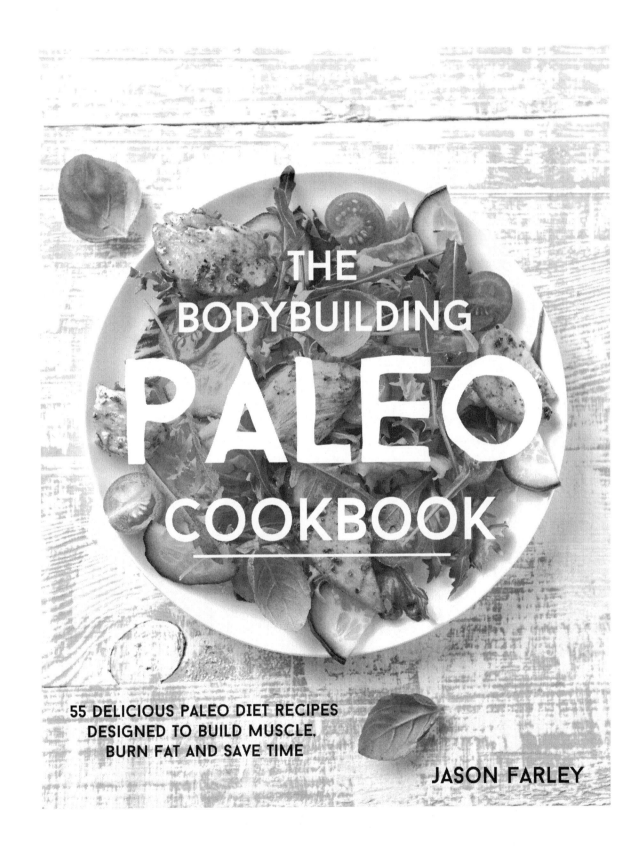

THE
Bodybuilding

PALEO

COOKBOOK

55 DELICIOUS PALEO DIET RECIPES
DESIGNED TO BUILD MUSCLE,
BURN FAT AND SAVE TIME

JASON FARLEY

If you want to learn how to create healthy, delicious and nutritious paleo meals that are specially designed to build muscle, burn fat and save time, then THE BODYBUILDING PALEO COOKBOOK is your answer!

Every serious athlete knows that your nutrition is the most crucial part of building a lean, muscular and strong physique and can either make or break the results you see in the gym. However keeping to a paleo diet while training can be extremely difficult as so many foods are just off limits. This can make things really tough, especially when you need to get in a certain amount of calories and fuel your demanding workouts in the gym!

And lets face it…

Most Paleo recipes are just downright bland and boring!

With The Bodybuilding Paleo Cookbook, you'll never have to be frustrated with your paleo diet again. You'll learn how to cook tasty, quick and easy paleo meals that will build quality lean muscle mass, burn fat fast and save time. Every recipe included in this cookbook has been meticulous designed with the right macronutrient profile (protein, fats & carbs) to ensure that you reach your training goals!

And in case you were wondering, these recipes aren't just a slight upgrade to the standard paleo recipes like you'd find in most other cookbooks. These recipes are so delicious that you won't miss "regular" meals!

The Bodybuilding Paleo Cookbook includes…

• 7 mouth-watering breakfast meals like my Warrior Steak and Egg Supreme, Caveman Red Pepper Chicken Omelette, Action Avocado and Bacon Boost and Spiced Pumpkin Pancakes. They will kick-start your engine and ensure you start off the day as you mean to go on!

• 10 succulent and delicious chicken and poultry recipes like my Sweet Honey Chicken, Super Sticky Chicken Clubs and Grilled Chicken Kebabs. Say bye bye to boiled bland chicken. These meals will ensure that your body has no choice but to burn fat and build muscle!

And much, much more…

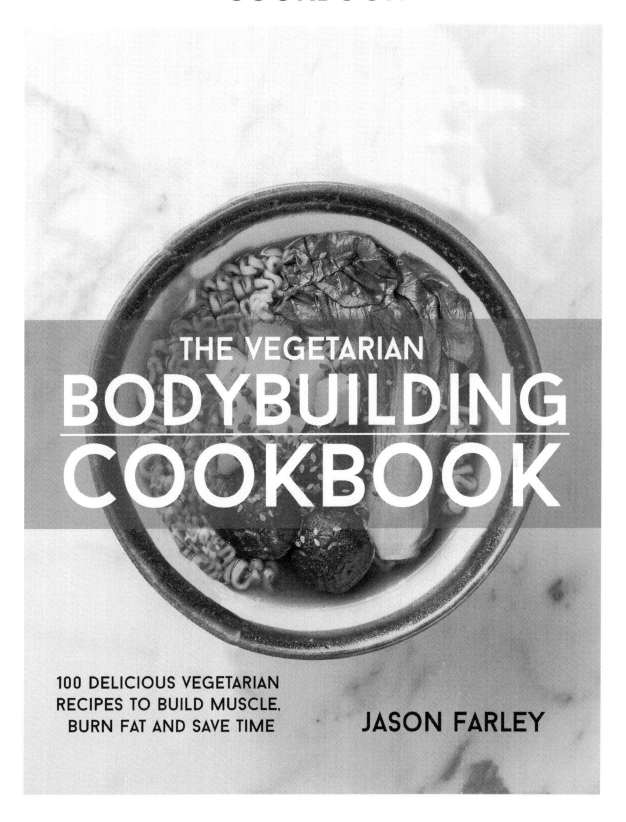

THE VEGETARIAN BODYBUILDING COOKBOOK

100 DELICIOUS VEGETARIAN RECIPES TO BUILD MUSCLE, BURN FAT AND SAVE TIME

JASON FARLEY

If you want to learn how to create healthy, delicious and nutritious vegetarian meals that are specially designed to build muscle, burn fat and save time, then THE VEGETARIAN BODYBUILDING COOKBOOK is your answer!

Every serious athlete knows that your nutrition is the most crucial part of building a lean, muscular and strong physique and can either make or break the results you see in the gym. However building muscle on a vegetarian diet can be more difficult as many foods are off limits. This can make things really tough, especially when you need to get in a certain amount of calories and fuel your demanding workouts in the gym!

And lets face it…

Most Vegetarian bodybuilding recipes are just downright bland and boring!

With The Vegetarian Bodybuilding Cookbook, you'll never have to be frustrated with your diet again. You'll learn how to cook healthy, tasty, quick and easy meals that will build quality lean muscle mass, burn fat fast and won't cost you an arm and a leg!

And these recipes aren't just a slight upgrade to familiar bodybuilding meals like you'd find in most health and fitness cookbooks. These recipes are so delicious your taste buds will believe you're in a 5 star restaurant!

The Vegetarian Bodybuilding Cookbook includes…

• 19 mouth-watering breakfast meals like my Muscle Fruit & Nut cereal , Lean & Mean Veggie Burger, Oat Muscle Mush and Brawny Veggie Sausage Club. They will kick-start your engine and ensure you start off the day as you mean to go on!

• 20 succulent and delicious entrees recipes like my Veggie Brawn Burger, Speedy Black Bean Surprise, Brawny Veg Lasagna, Tofu Lettuce Wraps and Feta & Brawny Barley Stuffed Portabellas. These meals will ensure that your body has no choice but to burn fat and build muscle!

• 19 gourmet snacks like my Muscle Feta Cheese & Olives, Quick Fix Roasted Beans, Protein Packed Latte and Sweet Potato Wedges.

• 13 tasty and nutritious sides like my Brawny Guacamole Hummus, Kale dip,

7645664R00149

Printed in Germany
by Amazon Distribution
GmbH, Leipzig